HEALTHCARE

LEADERSHIP

EXCELLENCE

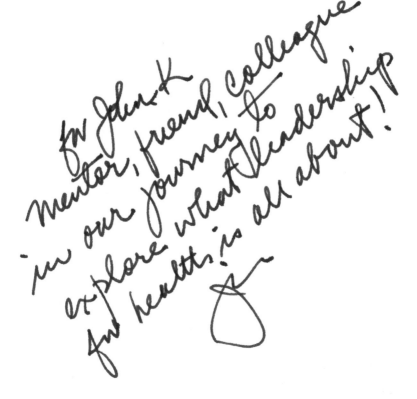

for John K
mentor, friend, colleague
- in our journey to
explore what leadership
for health, is all about!

HEALTHCARE

LEADERSHIP EXCELLENCE

Creating a Career of Impact

JAMES A. RICE & FRANKIE PERRY

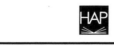

ACHE Management Series

Your board, staff, or clients may also benefit from this book's insight. For more information on quantity discounts, contact the Health Administration Press Marketing Manager at (312) 424–9470.

17   16   15   14   13   5   4   3   2   1

Library of Congress Cataloging-in-Publication Data
Rice, James A.
  Healthcare leadership excellence : creating a career of impact / James A. Rice and Frankie Perry.
     p. cm.
  Includes bibliographical references and index.
  ISBN 978-1-56793-474-8 (alk. paper)
  1. Health services administration–United States. 2. Leadership–United States. 3. Business etiquette. I. Perry, Frankie. II. Title.
  RA971.R52 2012
  362.1068–dc23
                    2012020606

The paper used in this publication meets the minimum requirements of American National Standard for Information Sciences—Permanence of Paper for Printed Library Materials, ANSI Z39.48-1984. ♾™

Acquisitions editor: Carrie McDonald; Project manager: Joyce Dunne; Cover designer: Marisa Jackson; Layout: Fine Print, Ltd.

Found an error or a typo? We want to know! Please e-mail it to hap1@ache.org, and put "Book Error" in the subject line.

For photocopying and copyright information, please contact Copyright Clearance Center at www.copyright.com or at (978) 750–8400.

  Health Administration Press
  A division of the Foundation of the American
     College of Healthcare Executives
  One North Franklin Street, Suite 1700
  Chicago, IL 60606–3529
  (312) 424–2800

A legacy is defined as something handed down
from ancestor or predecessor.
A leadership legacy is the knowledge, stories,
experiences, and lessons passed on to others
by someone in a position of authority or power.
It is a memorable impact that is embedded
into the lives of others.

—*Lynda McDermott,*
"What Will Be Your Leadership Legacy?"

When you die they'll indicate on your tomb
the year of your birth and the year of your death
separated by a dash (1960–2020).
The dash is your life. What you did. How you lived.
Whose life you touched. The legacy you left behind.
The more purposefully engaged you are in helping others,
the deeper and finer and more memorable is your dash.

—*Dr. Nido Qubein,*
"Why It Is Important to Leave a Legacy"

If your actions create a legacy that inspires others
to dream more, learn more, do more and become more,
then, you are an excellent leader.

—*Dolly Parton*

Contents

Foreword

WHAT KIND OF legacy will you leave when you reach the sunset of your career and look back? One of the benchmarks I use is the collection of notes I have received from colleagues, physicians, patients, and employees throughout the years.

Here are some of the notes that I treasure:

Feedback from a faculty member of a leadership academy I started 12 years ago:

> Ten years ago, Leadership Academy had the promise of being a very special and unique leadership development program, fueled by your passion to teach and your vision of growing future generations of leaders who embraced your values of integrity, transparency, accountability, and teamwork. You described each year's class and the growing alumni ranks as your "agents of culture change"—the emerging leaders who would see beyond the silos of individual operating units to the power of a unified organization. Thank you for the opportunity to learn about leadership along with each class and to profoundly understand that it is always, always about the people.

A pharmacy employee's response to a daily blog describing the experiences of a medical response team sent by Scripps Health, San Diego, to Houston after Hurricane Katrina:

> I am so touched by the stories you are sharing with those of us back here in San Diego. It brings tears to my eyes every time I read how one of our fellow staff are affected by these people that have so much despair in their life. We can only imagine what it is

like. The media always seems to put some kind of political spin on everything which makes it difficult to comprehend. Please continue to send your daily updates of what it is really like. It brings us all closer together. It's wonderful that our organization is able to participate in this relief process. Let everyone know how proud we are to know our organization has such dedicated, compassionate people who have put their own lives on hold for a period of time in order to help those in such dire need. Thank you again for your communication with us.

A physician's response to a blog describing the experiences of the medical response team deployed by Scripps Health to Haiti after the 2010 earthquake:

I am an internist and have been here [at Scripps] for 17 years. The journal from the field that you send us each day is so moving that my eyes tear up every time I read it. I have to catch my breath before I can go see my next patient. I read your experiences to my family and friends and my children, at 10 and 12 years old, are so inspired, they too want to be on the next plane to Haiti. I have done medical work in other countries and know the fulfillment one gets from helping those in need. I love that feeling. Those of us at home are cheering for you, and we are proud of you. We hope you stay safe, and healthy, and heal many.

Legacy is a concept that I never gave much thought to in my early years in management, and though I suspect very few people do, looking back, I see that legacy is one of the most important dynamics for a leader to consider.

When I completed graduate school, my goal was simply to find a job—a leadership position in a quality organization that might offer me a good career and an opportunity for future advancement. I knew that I loved healthcare operations, and maybe, if I was successful, I might ultimately become a chief operating officer at some point in my career.

Well, as I often tell students and others who come to visit with me, I "fell up" in my career, and I went far beyond my original career goals.

Over the years, I began to think less about my career track and more about the difference I was—or was not—making in my work and in my life. It struck me that I was certainly not solely responsible for my success; instead, it was the people who worked with and for me who had vaulted me to success. I realized it was important for me to dedicate more of my time and energy to finding ways to make it better for those who had made it better for me. And once I became a CEO, I realized that I was responsible for a legacy that spanned many areas and covered numerous stakeholders—patients, the organization, the community, and my profession—and wondered what a positive legacy would look like in these areas.

Jim Rice and Frankie Perry have written a unique leadership book exploring the concept of legacy. Frankly, I wish this book had been available in the early stages of my career, as legacy is created over the entirety of one's career, not a concept we contemplate only when we enter its final stages. Legacy should be a consideration when we select an organization for which to work as well as when we make decisions that affect our patients, staff, physicians, and community. Most importantly, it should be a journey of events we manage proactively rather than occurrences we just let happen. The decisions we make and the actions we take every day not only will follow us during our entire career but, taken jointly, will comprise what will be our legacy.

This foreword began with some notes that are very important to me. Their words give me a sense of the legacy I might be leaving. I conclude with one more:

I will never forget the first day of the Leadership Academy. We were all asked to share something about ourselves. Each person was incredibly genuine when they spoke. As it moved from one person to the next around the table, I could not help but reflect that this experience would be life changing for me. As it moved around the table getting closer and closer to me, I began to feel something inside that I really cannot explain. When my turn came, I began to share, and in so doing, was brought to tears because I was so moved by what I knew would be a great moment in my life for personal growth. On the one hand, I was embarrassed for becoming emotional, yet on the other hand, I felt total acceptance from Chris and my peers. As I journeyed through the year, I began to see all of my many flaws and how if I would step back and acknowledge them, I could grow and become a more effective leader. The greatest lessons came from Chris. Not so much in what he said, but his transparency and lead by example approach. I remember him acknowledging weakness and his dependence on surrounding himself with the best people. I will cherish the growth I experienced, the friendships made, and the many reflective notes written to memorialize all of the special moments in which my eyes were opened to yet another area of my life that I previously had not seen.

Enjoy the book, as well as the people you will touch and the legacy you will leave.

Chris D. Van Gorder, FACHE
President and CEO
Scripps Health

Preface

MORE THAN 20 years ago in a Budapest café, a senior Ministry of Health leader asked me, "Do you know the difference between hospital leaders in the former Soviet Union and yours in the United States? Yours are optimistic about the future and worry about their legacy. Ours are pessimistic about the future and don't think about a legacy." Though perhaps a bit cynical, that sentiment planted a seed of curiosity that grew into this text.

Over the past two decades, as we have aged, we have watched and listened to leaders in more than 30 countries, across industries, and from both for-profit and not-for-profit enterprises. We have explored questions about legacy, jobs that matter, and careers of impact. The following five recurring questions have guided these conversations:

1. Do healthcare leaders think about their legacy, and if so, how do they seek to build and leave behind a positive legacy?
2. How do they describe a career that has made a positive difference?
3. What legacy do they hope to leave with
   —their employers,
   —their community,
   —their industry, and
   —their family?
4. How can a healthcare leader be more intentional about building and nurturing a legacy?

5. Which practical strategies can a leader in the hospital and healthcare sector use to improve his or her chances for a career of impact?

This book explores answers to these questions and offers insights targeted not just to early careerists but also to mid- and late careerists refining their careers.

Twenty-one senior leaders from the US hospital and healthcare sector were interviewed regarding their career plans and progression in careers of impact. Scores of studies were examined about leadership and a leader's legacy. The result is a distillation of ideas that we hope will help you plot your legacy road map and ignite your and your colleagues' excitement about, and effectiveness in, shaping your journey to a legacy you are proud of for your organization, your community, our field, and your family.

James A. Rice, 2011

WHEN WE THINK of *legacy,* we think of leaving a legacy. And of course, we all want to be well remembered when we are gone and to have made a significant contribution while we were here. But rather than leaving a legacy, our challenge to you in this book is to *live a legacy.* You need to "live" leadership that makes a difference and that results in a career of impact. This kind of legacy is built day by day—not at the end of your career, or in the middle—but from the very beginning and throughout your professional journey.

Certain characteristics are requisite building blocks for creating a strong leadership foundation. These building blocks are the focus of Part II of this book.

But having this foundation in place is only the beginning. A career of impact must be sustainable and live on through the accomplishments and contributions of others who have benefited from the experiences and wisdom of the leader. This legacy of perpetuity only happens when certain leadership characteristics are so ingrained within the leader that they become a consistent way of life. Not the least of these is an unselfish intellectual generosity—a sharing of knowledge and insights that is motivated by a genuine desire to help others achieve personal and organizational success and not intended to garner recognition or reward for the leader. Such are the contributions of the leaders interviewed here, whose comments are integrated throughout the chapters.

Leadership is a skill that can be consciously learned and developed. But we must be mindful of the essential leadership characteristics and how we embody them; this process is the path to personal and spiritual growth. Self-reflection brings self-realization and the recognition that there is more to life than what we are doing. It is what we are being. In a recent interview, Neil Donald Walsh, author of *Conversations with God,* says authentic leaders must detach themselves from the outcome. Furthermore, they must develop the idea of themselves as compassionate, kind, honest, just, trustworthy, innovative, or another positive descriptor and then seek the experience of that idea. It is our hope that our readers will develop or enhance that idea of themselves as leaders and live into it.

WHO BENEFITS?

Leaders in healthcare provider organizations at all stages of their careers are encouraged to keep this book at hand on their shelves and use it as a catalyst to be more intentional about building a career of impact. It can serve as a resource to further enhance leadership skills and provide a ready reference for guiding careers in ways that you and those who work with you garner more rewards. It can be used for one's personal and professional development, as a teaching tool for those one mentors, and as a guide for staff development throughout the organization.

Healthcare managers entering the field will find it useful in charting their path in the early stages of their careers. It will influence how they look for jobs and the leadership skills they seek to develop, and it can make them more aware of the value of mentorship and more receptive to being mentored.

Mid-careerists will find it useful as a guide to assess the impact and value of their contributions at this stage of their careers. This assessment may motivate them to adjust their career path and focus on skill development and experiences that will achieve greater impact.

Executives in the pre-retirement and retirement years can use the text as a guide to evaluate their contributions and strategize ways to strengthen and enhance their legacy within the era of their encore performance.

At the end of each chapter, you will find three action steps to take now that will help mark the milestones along your journey to a career of impact. These are the kinds of actions that legacy leaders and those aspiring to high-performance leadership take as they live a leadership journey and create a legacy that matters.

Frankie Perry, 2011

Acknowledgments

THE HEALTHCARE LEADERS listed below were gracious with their time and insights as this book was being formed. Their wisdom and contributions to the endeavor and to our field are very much appreciated.

Brian Campion, MD, is senior fellow in healthcare leadership at Opus College of Business, University of St. Thomas, in Minneapolis.

Ed Dahlberg, LFACHE, is former president and CEO of St. Luke's Regional Medical Center in Boise, Idaho.

Thomas C. Dolan, PhD, FACHE, CAE, is president and CEO of the American College of Healthcare Executives in Chicago.

Martin L. "Chip" Doordan, LFACHE, is CEO emeritus at Anne Arundel Health System in Annapolis, Maryland.

David J. Fine, FACHE, is president and CEO of St. Luke's Episcopal Health System in Houston.

Patricia Gabow, MD, is CEO of Denver (Colorado) Health & Hospital Authority.

Patrick G. Hays, FACHE, is an advisor to management at the University of Southern California in Los Angeles.

Paul B. Hofmann, DrPH, FACHE, is president of Hofmann Healthcare Group in Moraga, California.

Stanley F. Hupfeld is chairman of INTEGRIS Family of Foundations at INTEGRIS Health in Oklahoma City.

John G. King, LFACHE, is president of John G. King Associates in Scottsdale, Arizona.

Lowell C. Kruse, LFACHE, is president and CEO emeritus at Heartland Health in St. Joseph, Missouri.

Stephanie S. McCutcheon, FACHE, is principal at McCutcheon and Co. in Pasadena, Maryland.

Stanley R. Nelson, LFACHE, is chairman of Scottsdale Institute in Minneapolis.

Kirk Oglesby is president emeritus of AnMed Health in Anderson, South Carolina.

Samuel L. Ross, MD, is CEO of Bon Secours Baltimore (Maryland) Health System.

Nancy M. Schlichting is CEO of Henry Ford Health System in Detroit.

William C. Schoenhard, FACHE, is deputy under secretary for Health Operations and Management at the US Department of Veterans Affairs in Washington, D.C.

Harvey Smith is president and CEO of Pacific Medical Centers in Seattle.

Mark R. Tolosky, JD, FACHE, is president and CEO of Baystate Health in Springfield, Massachusetts.

Gail L. Warden, LFACHE, is president emeritus of Henry Ford Health System in Detroit.

Donald C. Wegmiller, FACHE, is vice chairman of Scottsdale Institute and chairman emeritus of Integrated Healthcare Strategies in Minneapolis.

Introduction

THE DECADE FROM 2011 to 2020 will see thousands of hospital and health system leaders transition into retirement or make career changes. Many of these leaders will not be prepared for these career shifts, and some have begun to wonder to what degree their careers have made a difference in the lives of their staff, their organizations, or their communities. In the dark of night they ask themselves variations on these questions: "Does my passing through this life matter?" and "Am I living a career of impact and significance or merely a loosely connected string of jobs?"

This book offers fresh insights into how healthcare leaders can improve their prospects of having a "career of impact." It distills wisdom and lessons from three sources:

1. Interviews with 21 respected hospital and healthcare leaders
2. A library of business texts on leadership and legacies
3. The extensive health-sector experiences of the authors

The purpose of this text is to encourage and motivate healthcare leaders to think beyond the pressing day-to-day challenges of their organizations and plan for their long-term professional life. It is written for those who wish to create a career of impact and to leave a meaningful legacy.

To help you begin—or continue—your legacy journey, we emphasize the importance of developing self-awareness, building essential skills, and instilling the attributes that produce leaders who make a difference. Toward that end, we present seven necessary building blocks for a career of impact. As you read about these, ask yourself where you need to focus more attention and how you can develop your personal road map to achieve this goal. The idea behind the road map is to guide hospital and health system leaders through three career eras: the early (first 10) years, the middle (approximately the next 20) years, and the later (last 20) years.

Insights gleaned from our interviews with prominent healthcare leaders complement the strategies discussed for creating the career-of-impact road map. Advice from these leaders tended to fall within three categories of legacy-leaving lessons—slow awakening, enlightened self-interest, and intentional initiatives—which correspond to the three career eras. We introduce each category in the following sections.

SLOW AWAKENING: THE EARLY YEARS

The healthcare leaders we interviewed concluded that they could have been more deliberate in developing and then following a career road map than they had been as early careerists. They note that a key activity is to listen to the call to plan for, rather than drift through, the early years of a career.

> "I never really thought much about 'a legacy'; I was just focused on doing my job."

> "I'm a physician. I drifted into my leadership roles with no plan and no clue. Thankfully, I had a mentor, but she didn't talk about 'legacy,' just smarter listening."

> "Legacy? In the early years, I was happy to have 'a job.' Then I wanted a 'fulfilling job.' Later in my career, I started to see the importance of helping 'others find a fulfilling job.'"

ENLIGHTENED SELF-INTEREST: THE MIDDLE YEARS

As these leaders progressed through their careers, they increasingly recognized the power of collaboration with others to serve patients and communities.

"I did not use the word *legacy*, but I finally started to wonder if all the long hours and bold projects really made any difference. Would my management matter?"

"My first embrace of anything like 'legacy thinking' was more about . . . [t]he more I help *them* succeed, the more I will be able to accomplish. Now that seems a bit self-centered, but thankfully, I matured to realize the unleashing of their talents helped us serve patients smarter, not just our egos or economics!"

"The older I get, the more sincere I get about leveraging my talents with, through, and for the enhanced talents of my staff. Together we do more, and leave more good for the organization's vitality, and for the communities we exist to serve."

INTENTIONAL INITIATIVES: THE LATER YEARS

But the real insights about practicing leadership that matters and ensuring a career of impact became clearer to our interviewed leaders in the twilight of their careers. Leadership that makes a difference is much more likely to occur as we learn to listen to and mentor those around us at work, at home, and in the community.

"I get it now; to leave a meaningful mark, I've had to intentionally raise the bar on my development of not just my own competencies but the effectiveness and engagement of leaders throughout the organization."

"The health sector will always be complex and changing. A lasting difference in the performance of large healthcare delivery organizations won't just happen by magic nor management. We need leaders who care about and catalyze the work of others. But that caring and catalyzing needs to be more carefully planned and implemented in a more disciplined way."

"Sustained performance that is continuously improved—that's what matters. To have a career of impact, we need to start sooner and be smarter, more supportive, and more systematic in the development of the leaders and staff around us."

In this book, we distill these leaders' journeys into a set of insights that can help you develop a sensible road map for achieving a satisfying and successful career. As you reflect on the three stages of your career, note where you are now and how best to implement your road map to a career of impact.

If you are in the *early years* of your career,

- develop a written plan that addresses each building block,
- stay current with the literature from the healthcare sector and the corporate world,
- emulate successful leaders,
- actively participate in continuing education and professional associations,
- seek out mentors and role models,
- develop a network of colleagues with whom you can share knowledge and experiences,
- be generous in sharing and enthusiastic about learning,
- practice leadership skills within your sphere of influence,
- learn what works and what may not,
- take advantage of resources available to you within and outside your organization,
- regularly revisit your road map,
- take time for self-reflection, and
- make adjustments as needed.

If you are in the *middle years* of your career and do not have a career plan, now is the time to

- build on your experiences;
- strengthen your leadership skills;
- develop a strategic plan for the remainder of your career;

- focus on putting those building blocks in place that need your attention;
- incorporate mentoring into your professional life, both as one being mentored and as one serving as a mentor to early careerists; and
- make continuing education, networking, and actively participating in your professional association a routine part of your professional life.

If you are in the *later years* of your career, you should be intentionally

- mentoring,
- building a pipeline of successors for each of your C-suite direct reports, and
- developing the competencies and confidence of your direct middle managers.

Furthermore, for later-career executives, now is the time to participate in conversations about career and retirement planning. These conversations should focus on five key questions:

Q1. Recognizing that your retirement could span 30 years (from age 65 to 95), how have you been exploring what you would love to do over the next 10 to 20 years—not just to leverage your friends, funds, and fun but to give back some time and talent to your community and the healthcare field?

Q2. Considering you have had staff help support your professional accomplishments and drive over the past ten years, who will provide the infrastructure and resources you and your spouse will need for your next decade of activities for such varied issues as the following:
- Continuous learning and intellectual growth?
- Time to reconnect and enhance undernourished exploration of family, friends, and faith?

- Regional and international travel?
- Consulting opportunities?
- Interim executive work assignments in healthcare or other segments of society?
- Personal health and fitness?
- Mentoring community and healthcare leaders and assisting organizations?

Q3. With the erosion of assets from the recession that began in 2008, how will you earn additional income and cover your health or disability insurance needs? Do you fully understand how much cash you will need every month to live comfortably as the cost of living, taxes, and insurance inevitably continue to rise?

Q4. Have you begun to develop a calendar of interactions, reflections, and analysis to define the legacy you will be leaving with your organization, industry, family, community, and friends? What eclectic readings have you planned to study to learn how other leaders contemplate their next 10 to 20 years of active retirement or a second or third career?

Q5. During the past few years, what activities and relationships have given you the most joy, sense of purpose, and pride of performance, and how will you ensure they continue or become enhanced?

Most executives will find no easy answers to these questions. But the process of exploring them may help you to continue along your road map to a career of impact.

Throughout a healthcare leader's career, perhaps the most difficult skill to learn is the ability to carve out the time for the self-reflection one requires to develop the self-awareness needed to experience a career that makes a difference. This book is intended to motivate healthcare leaders to make time for this essential building block to a career of impact. You do not need to be the CEO of a multi-institutional healthcare system, make a six-figure salary, employ a staff of thousands, or receive accolades and awards to create a career of impact. You do need to have left your sphere of influence a better place for having been there. Review and revisit the building blocks presented in this book, and share them with those you may be mentoring, as a guide to help you along the journey.

At the end of each chapter are three action steps to take now that will contribute to setting the building blocks. They are the kinds of actions that leaders and those aspiring to leadership take to create a legacy that matters.

PART I

The Leadership Challenge

CHAPTER 1

Leadership Clarity: Bedrock for Legacy Thinking

LEADERSHIP IS DEFINED by the ability to get needed work done with and through others. It is a group and team endeavor, not a solo performance. Leaders with an unfocused view of leadership rarely accomplish as much as those with a clear understanding of the broad set of knowledge, skills, and attitudes needed to inspire, mobilize, and guide diverse people and groups toward important purposes using sensible processes. These attributes for success are referred to as leadership competencies.

The National Health Service (NHS) in the United Kingdom has spent more than a decade developing an understanding of the leadership competencies essential for positive improvements in clinical outcomes, staff morale, and patient satisfaction (Exhibit 1.1). It learned that leadership is shaped by the presence of a handful of essential personal qualities:

- Self-belief
- Self-awareness
- Self-management
- Drive for improvement
- Personal integrity

The NHS's pursuit to define leadership competencies has culminated in the Leadership Framework (National Leadership Council

2010). This framework shows the relationship between the personal qualities mentioned above and the behaviors that characterize effective teamwork, which can lead to optimum service delivery. When one understands the nature of leadership competencies, one has a sense of leadership clarity.

Clarity about what you understand leadership to encompass, in turn, enhances legacy clarity. Industries other than healthcare have determined that a leader's legacy is reflected in the way people think,

Exhibit 1.1: The Leadership Framework

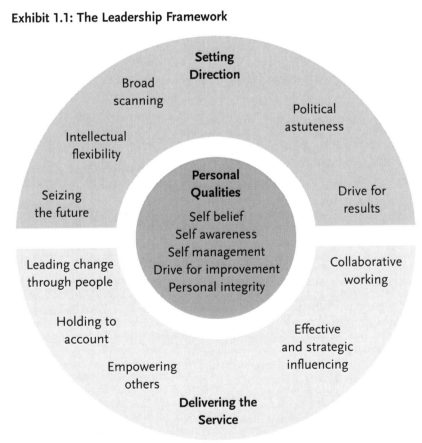

Source: Used with permission of the NHS Institute for Innovation & Improvement, London. www.leadershipacademy.nhs.uk/lf.

behave, approach work, and approach life as a result of having worked with that leader. It has little to do with one's abilities, measurable performance, or strategic savvy, and it has everything to do with who the leader is as a person at work and with the role he naturally plays, as opposed to his title and responsibilities.

We selected the 21 healthcare leaders interviewed for this book because they have demonstrated they are leaving a legacy of accomplishment and respect from colleagues in the field. Their reputations suggest they have evolved leadership competencies likely to yield a positive, lasting legacy. What can we learn from these leaders that might shape the legacy of others and the leadership development programs across the US health sector?

Most of the healthcare executives interviewed considered their career planning process and achievement of accomplishments to have evolved informally rather than intentionally. They cite a bit of good luck in attaining early job opportunities and good mentors. Several acknowledged their hard work, the influence of their mentors, and their advance planning as contributing to their leadership progression. While their style of career planning varied from accepting positions at organizations in which they had a good feeling about their boss or chairperson to deliberately targeting markets in which organizational growth was likely, several interviewed leaders admitted to encountering sleepless nights at those career junctures where they recognized the need to map out strategies to bond with physicians, board leaders, and philanthropists. Underlying that self-effacing sense of "serendipitous" good fortune, however, are invariably good preparation, an open mind, and an early curiosity about leadership competencies and leader role models. Clarity as to what one believes to be the attributes of effective leadership is the bedrock of legacy thinking. It is this clarity that we must seek if we are to hope for more intentional planning for our legacy.

Most healthcare executives think of legacy as a consideration that can wait until later in their career, at the edge of retirement; some do not think about legacy at all. Those leaders who do focus on their legacy in the midst of their career find they are better, more effective

> **Effective leaders love** asking challenging questions.
>
> They should also not be afraid to question with a beginner's mind and within the Buddhist admonition to be humble. You cannot be a great leader with only your intellect. The first key still is to listen, talk, and build a relationship; you care about what each person can contribute.
>
> I was unsophisticated about 'leadership' learning and initially not great at 'management.'
>
> —**Brian Campion**, MD

leaders today as a result. One's desired leadership legacy should be a catalyst for action rather than a conclusion considered after the career is over. This approach to a consideration of legacy is referred to as legacy thinking.

Maruca and Galford (2006) note the power inherent in sparking legacy thinking early in one's career. In their studies among college-level students they ask, "Are you on this planet to do something, or are you here just for something to do? If you're on this planet to do something, then what is it? What difference will you make? What will be your legacy?"

By asking ourselves how we as healthcare leaders want to be remembered, we plant the seeds for living our lives—not just our careers—as if we matter. By doing so, we offer up our unique legacy to those we live and work with. By clarifying that unique legacy, we are more likely to make the world we inhabit a better place than we found it.

Most healthcare leaders have not seriously considered these questions at any point in their life or career. When prompted to answer them, scores of senior healthcare executives we have interacted with affirm that the question, "What will be my legacy?" has neither a single answer nor a right answer. But asking the question and searching for clear answers help all of us recognize that along life's journey we will periodically struggle with determining the nature of the difference we hope to make and what activities matter most. We make choices at school, at work, at home, and in the community, and every choice forms part of the legacy we leave, however consciously or unconsciously we behave.

WHAT WILL YOUR LEADERSHIP LEGACY BE?

You might be the smartest CEO or most brilliant strategist ever employed by your hospital, but if you left tomorrow, what would you leave behind? What would the people with whom you have worked do differently because they worked with you?

Building your legacy requires development work in three crucial areas: competencies, trust, and self-reflection. First, you must hone your competencies as a healthcare leader. Next, you become a trusted adviser to others and then take on the role of trusted leader. Finally, as that trusted leader, you practice self-reflection, which allows you to not only cultivate your legacy for tomorrow but also ensure your effectiveness as a leader today.

Leaving Your Legacy, Making Your Mark

Individuals should think about legacy on their way into a position rather than on their way out of one. The following paragraphs introduce a number of activities we have found useful to healthcare executives in ensuring they forge the legacy vision they desire—one that will be most likely to reflect the obituary they hope will be written to commemorate them.

New Conversations on What Really Matters

Asking questions about legacy brings forward a central observation: Success in healthcare leadership is not

> **"I did not think much** about a legacy in early years. My whole career has been dictated by serendipity and good fortune.
>
> My leadership mark and successes have been shaped by people ranging from early football coaches to hospital executives who took a chance with me. These opportunities suggest to me the need to consider this counsel: love, learn, lead to leave a legacy.
>
> Great leaders help our staff to learn from diverse projects: from volunteer projects to book clubs to meaningful organizational projects.**"**
>
> **—Stanley F. Hupfeld**

measured only in numbers. Being a leader brings with it a responsibility to play a significant role in an endeavor that ultimately leaves families, communities, organizations, nations, the environment, and the world better than they are today. Such a role involves many activities, and not all of them can be quantified, but all should be explored. We propose crafting a leadership legacy road map to guide these conversations.

Conversations About Leadership

We can begin to achieve clarity about leadership that matters by examining the nature of leadership in other industries. LaFasto and Larson (2001) analyzed the responses of 6,000 team members from across public- and private-sector industries about the strengths and weaknesses of the members' team leaders. The comments go well beyond identifying the qualities of good or bad leaders to describe the specific leader behaviors team members find most helpful and most instructive. LaFasto and Larson (2001, 96) found that an effective leader takes six important actions:

1. Focuses on the goal
2. Ensures a collaborative climate
3. Builds confidence
4. Demonstrates sufficient technical know-how
5. Sets priorities
6. Manages performance

A leader who takes these key actions is committing to adopting the following behaviors, which serve as plot points on her legacy road map (LaFasto and Larson 2001, 147):

- Make performance expectations clear.
- Encourage the team to agree on a set of values that guides its performance.
- Ensure that rewards and incentives are aligned with achieving the team's goal.

- Assess the collaborative skills of team members as well as the results they achieve.
- Give useful, developmental feedback to team members.
- Be willing to confront and resolve issues associated with inadequate performance by team members.
- Recognize and reward superior performance.

These lists should merely serve as a guide. The essential ingredient in the leadership recipe is an element only you can provide: the essence of who you are (LaFasto and Larson 2001, 150).

> **Leaders I have respected try to be calm, self-effacing, with a** sincere commitment to the mission and vitality of the organization. They care more about people than things or rewards. They are truthful with colleagues/staff and show them they have confidence for them to grow.
>
> —Kirk Oglesby

Networking Matters

Scores of autobiographies and leadership studies have concluded that legacies, like the leaders who leave them, are born of a marriage between innate characteristics and lifelong learning. While the healthcare leaders interviewed for this book cited several examples of early invitations to lead scout groups, bands, family gatherings, and numerous school and church groups, they also acknowledged the contributions to their advancement of broad networking opportunities through

- mentors;
- thoughtful followers; and
- diverse and eclectic learning environments, including
  —graduate school,
  —professional associations, such as the American College of Healthcare Executives,

—collegial exchange networks, and

—mentoring from an effective member of the executive's health system board.

In addition, some organizations, such as Premier, VHA Inc., and Health Insights, encourage leaders to develop eclectic reading habits on leadership, governance, talent management, and teamwork— inside and outside of healthcare—to help spice up networking encounters with colleagues.

Values Matter

Healthcare leaders, including those featured in this book, are often quick to reminisce about how fascinated they once were that a career path in hospital and healthcare management could offer an integration of the disciplines of business with the "softer" side of caring for and serving others. Several of the leaders interviewed were initially interested in the field of medicine or in becoming a physician, and many cited parents and religion as early influences encouraging them to be open to a purpose beyond the self.

Legacy leaders are found in every walk of life, from the boardroom to the battlefield, from public service to private homes, neighborhoods, schools, and communities. They are found in the worn pages of history books and in the memories of those who have been touched by them, and they continue to inspire and influence present and future leaders. The hallmark of legacy in leadership is its power to influence others enough to cause change—a shift from unconsciously "doing" leadership to consciously *being* a leader. The best way to effect that influence is in person, by living your legacy today, not waiting for others to reflect on the past tomorrow.

Sandstrom and Smith (2008, 27) propose five interrelated roles that effective leaders may adopt to achieve a career of impact that brings about the leadership shift in others:

Role One: Holder of Vision and Values™
Role Two: Creator of Collaboration and Innovation™
Role Three: Influencer of Inspiration and Leadership™
Role Four: Advocator of Differences and Community™
Role Five: Calibrator of Responsibility and Accountability™

They emphasize that the first word in each title represents the *being* part of that leadership practice. Great leaders must be clear that they are, first and foremost, a holder, a creator, an influencer, an advocator, and a calibrator. In other words, the greatness resides in *who they are* first, and *what they do* second.

A person's actions are dictated by her character. Some people debate whether a leader is born or created. We believe both innate abilities and environmental learning are contributors. While leadership has its foundation in the core of the leader—who she is—this core nature can be shaped by and transformed through self-reflection and interaction with effective mentors.

IN SEARCH OF "LEVEL 5" LEADERS

One of the most striking insights brought forth during a forum convened by Witt/Kieffer (2007) was the way participants described ideal leaders. The attributes they focused on involve character and integrity and have little to do with technical skills.

Participants also stressed the importance of personal drive tempered by humility, reminiscent of Collins' (2001) definition of Level 5 leaders in his *Good to Great* model. According to Collins, a Level 5 leader builds enduring greatness through a paradoxical blend of personal humility and professional will. High performers channel their ego needs into the larger goal of building a great company, Collins says.

We consider a majority of the interviewed healthcare leaders to be Level 5 leaders. These executives expressed humility but conveyed the bold visions they built for their organizations and colleagues in clear, insightful terms. They partner with colleagues, boards, and physicians to develop comprehensive strategies for pursuing stretch performance objectives for themselves and their organizations. Not content to focus their insights and will on achieving accomplishments within their organizations alone, most of the interviewed leaders have been active in regional and national leadership roles to serve the industry and develop future leaders for a challenging future. Such leaders are more likely to leave lasting legacies and high-performing healthcare organizations than are leaders who fall elsewhere along the spectrum of leadership.

A LEGACY-LEAVING LEADER

Leadership clarity is achievable if your legacy road map is built on the following leader attributes (adapted from Kouzes and Posner 2006, 49):

- Knows where he or she is going, why he or she is going there, and how to get there
- Looks for the best in those he or she serves
- Knows how to lead without being dictatorial; exhibits humility
- Does not look for or require kudos
- Considers leadership to be an opportunity to serve
- Learns to listen and listens to learn
- Has courageous conversations with ally and opponent alike
- Manages time, money, and resources as a good steward
- Has his or her head in the clouds but his or her feet on the ground

We all need to find our voice and use it to fulfill our life's passions, purpose, posture, and position to leave a legacy of leadership. Clarify your leadership voice and your gifts, and use them to develop those around you. The bedrock for legacy thinking is a solid appreciation for providing selfless service to earn followers with your inspiring vision, challenging expectations, passionate mentoring, and continuous pursuit of personal development.

THREE KEY ACTIONS TO HARDWIRE LEADERSHIP CLARITY INTO YOUR LEGACY ROAD MAP

Action 1: Explore and master leadership models from diverse resources, including distant sources such as the UK's National Health Service.

Action 2: Define your own set of leadership competencies that will drive your personal development and your mentoring of others, and place them in your personal digital assistant you transfer from smart phone to smart phone. You can refine the list periodically throughout your career.

Action 3: Draft your obituary in an upbeat and light-hearted style to reflect a career you would be proud to celebrate with those who mentored you.

PART II

Building Blocks for a Career of Impact

CHAPTER 2

Self-Reflection and Awareness

WE HAVE FOUND that a great leader is self-aware. One of the essential traits of legacy leaders is authenticity to self (George 2003, 11). The key to developing authenticity is a sense of self-awareness, which begins early in a career. This chapter expands on the concepts of self-reflection and self-awareness, including how to approach them and how to develop an organization-wide culture in which others can nurture their own authentic self.

> **"Self-assessment is key, as is a recognition [that], to be effective,** you are not going to get approval from everyone.**"**
>
> **—Harvey Smith**

WHY BE SELF-REFLECTIVE?

Effective leaders are willing to step back from situations and consider which style of leadership, strategic thinking tactic, means of engaging staff and colleagues in situation analysis, approach to defining the problem, or method of problem solving is most appropriate for each. They must also understand how to balance the three Ls—listening, learning, and leading—for each situation, a skill that significantly enhances their own and their leadership team's effectiveness. To gain this understanding, think about—that is, reflect on—your words, expressions, actions, and leadership style; your career planning; and your approach to team development.

Healthcare leaders are watched closely by colleagues and staff for signals about expected and acceptable behavior. If leaders want high-performance teams, they need to model desired behaviors, such as

- a passion to seek continuous improvement;
- a desire to serve patients, physicians, and purchasers with superior value;
- a willingness to engage and empower others; and
- an excitement to pursue innovation through active listening to the experiences and ideas of eclectic and diverse staff and stakeholders.

HOW TO BE SELF-REFLECTIVE

Our work in physician leadership development suggests that physicians have particular difficulty being self-aware or engaging in self-reflective analysis of how their interactions in various group settings are perceived. Physicians are acculturated in an environment characterized by individual competition to secure favored entry into medical school, internships, and residencies, and their training celebrates the value and expectation of self-reliant and individualistic decision making under time and data constraints. They are often surprised to learn in 360-degree assessments that they are perceived as autocratic, unwilling to consider the insights of others, and ineffective in group decision making.

Brian Campion, MD, a respected physician executive and cofounder of the successful Physician Leadership College at St. Thomas University in Minneapolis, has concluded that clinical leaders can most rapidly advance their career effectiveness by mastering active listening and the art and science of asking thoughtful questions. We refer to this skill as the Q factor. Leaders who have mastered the Q factor ask questions that cannot be answered by yes

❝It's a brand new year, and your major focus is most likely on next year's business plan and how you are going to achieve the goals and objectives you have set for the healthcare enterprise. This thought process focuses predominantly on business issues, external influences, strategy, and keeping your team focused on success.

But what about you? What are your personal plans as a leader for today and beyond? What are you doing to improve the impact you have on people? Who is responsible for your personal growth and success?

Effective leaders love engaging in meaningful dialogues and asking challenging questions.

They should also not be afraid to question with a beginner's mind and within the Buddhist admonition to be humble. You cannot be a great leader with only your intellect. The first key still is to listen, talk, and build a relationship; you care about what each person can contribute.

I was unsophisticated about 'leadership' learning and initially not great at 'management,' but several patient mentors moved me along the path. I have tried to do the same with my colleagues and staff.❞

—Brian Campion, MD

or no but that begin with or use phrases such as "Why are we . . . ?" "How else could we . . . ?" "When should we . . . ?" "What if we did it this way?" or "What are the risks of doing/not doing this?"

Excellent leaders tell us they are always ready to pursue alternate answers and not be content with conventional wisdom or with platitudes offered by insincere or solicitous subordinates. Furthermore, not only do effective leaders ask staff and colleagues Q factor questions, but they also ask similar questions of themselves, frequently and objectively.

The skill of asking good questions can be invaluable, as it forces us to wrestle with uncomfortable issues or provocative new perspectives. When the question is about your own performance, however, being objective about negative feedback may be difficult. When you show that you are open to all types of feedback, you demonstrate self-awareness and the willingness to learn. Bill George (www.billgeorge.org/page/true-north-groups) has observed that the essence of leadership comes not from having predefined characteristics. Rather, it comes from knowing yourself—your strengths and weaknesses—by understanding your unique life story and the challenges you have experienced.

Legacy leaders do not fear asking questions—they "learn to listen, and listen to learn," and they create a culture in their teams and organizations that encourages and enables key questions to be asked about the following types of issues:

- Confronting assumptions and mind-sets that filter our interpretation of situations, problem definitions, and problem solutions
- Identifying stakeholders who are most important to ask questions of and listen to
- Developing a shared commitment to create and nurture risk-free and blame-free zones in which colleagues and staff can offer candid views of the group's, their own, and the leader's effectiveness, strengths, and weaknesses

A culture that exhibits a high Q factor is also one of maturity. It serves as a setting for emotionally mature leaders, followers, and collaborators; these participants have high emotional intelligence (EQ) (Goleman 1992).

Following Goleman's EQ model helps healthcare leaders to master four competencies:

1. Self-awareness—the ability to read one's emotions and recognize their impact while using gut feelings to guide decisions
2. Self-management—the ability to control one's emotions and impulses and adapt to changing circumstances
3. Social awareness—the ability to sense, understand, and react to others' emotions while comprehending the importance of interactions we have in our various networks of colleagues, friends, and family members

4. Relationship management—the ability to inspire, influence, and develop others while managing conflict

EQ is discussed further in Chapter 8 in relation to developing a celebration culture.

An entire industry of assessment tools, executive coaches, and talent management firms has been spawned by the recognition that effective leaders and effective careers are rarely possible without (1) objective analysis and comparison of one's behaviors to evidence-based norms and (2) willingness to be receptive to the opinions of others. While self-awareness is among the least-discussed leadership competencies, it may be one of the most valuable (Musselwhite 2007).

Self-awareness reflects a willingness and an ability to objectively assess ourselves as if we were a wise and experienced friend evaluating our strengths and weaknesses. Objective self-evaluation covers dimensions such as the following:

- Appearance
- Language
- Moral values
- Active listening
- Integrity
- Open consideration of new and perhaps unpopular ideas or beliefs
- Sharing of credit and power
- Humility
- Engagement and empowerment of others

This self-evaluation can, and often should, allow you to reach the conclusion that you need to exhibit behaviors and perform actions appropriate for the social or organizational situation.

Many male leaders assume that their effectiveness must be shaped by an authoritarian or even autocratic management style. We disagree with this position and believe women leaders of the future are more likely to be successful among knowledge workers because they are more receptive to and accommodating of alternate ideas and approaches in general than are their male counterparts.

In the rapidly changing environment healthcare leaders face, many have adopted the mind-set that they are required to know everything. They fear people will not follow if they admit they do not have all the answers; any apparent vulnerability could diminish their effectiveness as leaders.

In fact, however, our experience with healthcare managers young and old indicates the opposite is true, especially for those who work in competitive markets with interdisciplinary teams that recognize the power of diverse perspectives and experiences.

Legacy leaders acknowledge their weaknesses and appreciate that those weaknesses will be seen by others. The person who tries to hide weakness actually highlights it, creating the perception that he lacks integrity (Musselwhite 2007).

To promote personal growth, healthcare leaders should regularly engage in self-analysis and reflection. They may begin the process by asking the following questions:

- What do I want physicians to say about me as an individual?
- What do I hope my grandchildren say about my accomplishments as a leader?
- What do I want my leadership legacy to be?
- What level of curiosity for innovation and excellence will I nurture in my employees?
- Am I an effective mentor? (See Chapter 5 for more about mentoring and legacy leadership.)

In short, how do you create a leadership legacy you can be proud of, one that speaks volumes about who you are and what you are accomplishing? Several of the healthcare leaders interviewed for this book suggest that the process begins by taking an inventory of your personal values (make sure you clearly distinguish your personal values from your business values in this exercise).

When reflecting about their careers, the 21 interviewed leaders each observed that a major portion of one's legacy road map is facing the challenge of creating balance in one's life. Achieving life balance allows you to embrace the expenditure of quality time on the five "F" priorities—family, friends, faith, fun, and fitness—as well as the overheralded three Fs of fiduciary, finances, and fame. Several of these executives acknowledge that finding a work–life balance with their family was not recognized as essential early enough in their careers to be fully accomplished. Once you understand and are willing to practice the concept of balance, they note, it comes more easily.

Your personal values platform serves as the basis for the business portion of your legacy, as demonstrated by your personal vision and mission. Your chosen vision and mission should reflect your passion, what you expect to accomplish, and how you will accomplish it. Your personal vision and mission are the foundation of your legacy.

As mentioned earlier, healthcare leaders often begin to consider the impact of their leadership when they are about to retire or moving to a senior-level job in another organization. They should not wait for these milestones to occur but should instead begin to look forward as soon as they enter the profession.

When looking forward, legacy healthcare leaders aim to achieve success in terms of organizational and personal performance. They hope to receive positive recognition for their efforts by the individuals they work with directly and indirectly. Kouzes and Posner (2006, 3), however, observe that being self-absorbed in one's legacy runs counter to the notion that leaders are selfless. By being more intentional about mapping your career plans, you can enhance the accomplishments of your career and the careers of those around you without having to indulge in self-absorbing, praise-seeking behavior.

Self-confidence and self-esteem pose different considerations than selfish pursuit of legacy. These two ingredients are necessary to make a positive difference, and they can encourage healthcare leaders to continuously explore a sense of self and self-worth that transcends the job or even the career. While necessary, however, self-confidence and self-esteem are not sufficient to build a career of impact. The leaders we spoke with are well aware that success cannot be achieved in a vacuum. They needed support along the way—financial, psychological, and other forms of assistance. They attracted this support through the intensity of their convictions and their awareness of the impressions they made on others. They became effective leaders because people believed in them, and people believed in them because they believed in themselves (Watson 2001, vii–ix).

THREE KEY ACTIONS TO HARDWIRE SELF-REFLECTION INTO YOUR LEGACY ROAD MAP

Action 1:   Boldly define your desired career goals using the SMART goal-setting format (they should be specific, measurable, attainable, realistic, and timely). Conduct a candid assessment of your values that will serve as a guide for your journey to achieve these goals.

Action 2:   Explore the art and science of the Q factor by asking questions that help clarify your values. These questions will guide your journey into a career of impact.

Action 3:   Take a risk: Post your values in a public forum, and invite your staff and colleagues to discuss yours and define their own. Dialogues stimulated by self-awareness yield positive career plans.

CHAPTER 3

Integrity and Character

A PAIR OF leadership attributes that are often overlooked or relegated to secondary importance are character and integrity. Leadership failures of industry titans, business owners, politicians, and yes, healthcare executives are often failures of character.

It follows, then, that leaving a positive legacy requires leading a life and career of high integrity. But few business schools and academic institutions teach values as a part of leadership development. Ethics courses are often theoretical and seem far removed from the realities of the workplace; in addition, faculty may assume that students are already ethical. But even if that assumption is accurate, the ethical nature of students does not automatically translate to ethics practiced in the office setting. Academic programs have failed to recognize the need for focused study in this arena, including the ways in which the changing healthcare environment influences values (George 2003, 21).

A highly reputable publisher recently advised an author to delete the word *ethics* from the title of his work because, he said, "Everyone thinks they are ethical." Certainly, no one will admit to being unethical, and few will admit they may benefit from guidance in the ethics discipline. Yet we are reminded daily of the misdeeds of prominent political, corporate, and even religious leaders who have violated standards of acceptable behavior. Regardless of the good they may have accomplished in their careers, it is the breach of character, the lack of integrity, the scandal that will be remembered.

It is said that Arthur Andersen lost its excellent reputation established over 50 years in one day following the Enron debacle (George 2003, 75).

The moral and cultural shifts in US society and the ever-increasing complexity of healthcare delivery have complicated executives' decision-making process. Healthcare leaders are especially challenged to feel confident that they are making ethically responsible decisions. While healthcare can be considered a microcosm of society in some ways, the level of complexity in healthcare management is disproportionately high compared to that of the corporate world in general. Advances in medical technology, the labyrinth of healthcare financing and reimbursement, the reform mandate, complex business transactions, increasing consumer expectations, public scrutiny, legislative requirements, and the proliferation of socioeconomic factors exacerbating health problems for certain populations are just some of the issues that complicate healthcare management as a context in which a leader explores his character development. Healthcare managers frequently find themselves in uncharted waters where the ethical rules may be unclear. Globalization and the acceleration of cross-cultural perceptions on acceptable behavior add yet another level of uncertainty for US healthcare leaders engaged internationally.

Real-life ethical dilemmas rarely involve a single ethical issue to resolve. More often, a number of issues converge, with many stakeholders, carrying diverse sets of values, clamoring for the chance to influence the outcome. Ambiguities abound. Often the matter is not simply a case of right or wrong, but a case of two competing "right" decisions with different outcomes.

Building character that ensures a career of impact and promises a legacy our families will be proud of is not easy. In ethical dilemmas,

"Organizational culture always has been and always will be largely determined for better or for worse by the CEO."

—**Paul B. Hofmann**, DrPH, FACHE

we often find ourselves on that "slippery slope," and character is what determines whether we slip and how far we slide.

CHARACTER AT THE CENTER OF LEADERSHIP

Consider General Norman Schwarzkopf's caution: "Leadership is a potent combination of strategy and character. But if you must be without one, be without strategy." Zenger and Folkman (2002, 12), in their book *The Extraordinary Leader: Turning Good Managers into Great Leaders,* report that "character is at the center of leadership" and is "the core of all leadership effectiveness." Furthermore, they write, "The impact that a leader has on others is the direct expression of the character of the individual and is the window by which others understand the character of the individual" (Zenger and Folkman 2002, 14). They describe what they consider to be fatal flaws that impair leadership capabilities. A person who is not honorable, does not keep promises, does not tell the truth, and places personal gain above the interests of the organization cannot hope to achieve true leadership status (Zenger and Folkman 2002, 24).

Some authors maintain that character is synonymous with leadership. As cited by Zenger and Folkman (2002, 55), respected management authority Max DePree has "equated leadership with personal character." Jim Shaffer has determined that "leadership is defined by telling the truth," and Stephen Covey stresses the "importance of leaders following principles in daily behavior" (quoted in Zenger and Folkman 2002, 56). Kouzes and Posner (1993, 14) have "defined personal credibility as the foundation of all leadership"; they describe a credible person as one who is honest, trustworthy, competent, and inspiring, and they propose that "Leadership is a relationship with credibility as the cornerstone."

In their research regarding the characteristics of admired leaders, Kouzes and Posner (1993, 15, 23) found that honesty was rated as the most important determinant regardless of country, region, or type of organization. They cite survey after survey ranking integrity as the number one attribute needed by great leaders—whether those surveyed were top executives or office workers. Above all, note Kouzes and Posner, leaders must be trusted. If they are not, nothing they say will be believable and they will soon lose their stature as a leader. As a result, employees and others will be reluctant to follow them.

These findings are interesting, given that ethics continuing education rarely attracts the participants that other, more technical skill–based programs do and given that prominent executives are often lauded for their financial performance, negotiating skills, ability to turn around failing organizations—success sometimes attained through questionable ethical practices. Do we acknowledge the value of integrity in leaders, especially those to whom we report, but fail to make ethics a priority in our professional development and that of our staff? Effective leaders recognize the merit of making ethics education and ethical standards priorities throughout the organization.

Conventional wisdom tells us that management is not a popularity contest, and while that maxim is true, healthcare leaders must earn the respect and admiration of employees, board members, physician colleagues, and community leaders if those stakeholders are to be loyal and committed to the organization (Kouzes and Posner 1993, 31).

Finally, a leader's character directly affects her organization's results. If people perceive the leader to be motivated by personal rewards rather than organizational or team success, they are less motivated to help achieve desired goals (Zenger and Folkman 2002, 80).

BARRIERS TO ETHICAL DECISION MAKING— SEVEN PITFALLS TO AVOID

If we agree with the research findings that character is the critical attribute for authentic leadership, and assuming we want to leave a legacy of high regard, why is integrity difficult to build or maintain? What are the barriers to ethical decision making? The following are seven pitfalls to avoid in building a legacy of integrity.

Pitfalls to Ethics

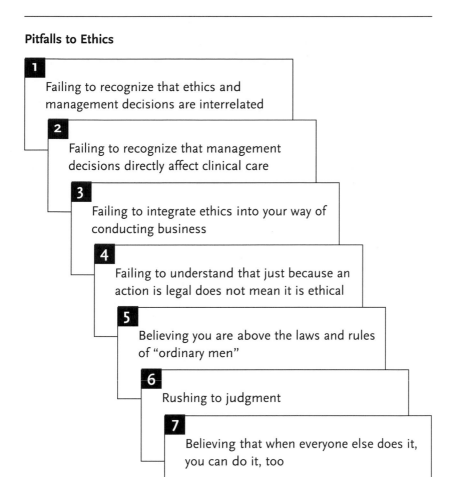

1 Failing to recognize that ethics and management decisions are interrelated

2 Failing to recognize that management decisions directly affect clinical care

3 Failing to integrate ethics into your way of conducting business

4 Failing to understand that just because an action is legal does not mean it is ethical

5 Believing you are above the laws and rules of "ordinary men"

6 Rushing to judgment

7 Believing that when everyone else does it, you can do it, too

Pitfall 1: Failing to Recognize That Ethics and Management Decisions Are Interrelated

A common mistake among leaders and managers is failing to recognize the interrelatedness of ethics and management decisions (Exhibit 3.1). They may relegate ethics to secondary importance or, worse, completely ignore it while management decisions are made on the sole basis of financial data, market share, and other bottom-line considerations. When ethical issues related to management decisions are unexamined or are cast aside as irrelevant, detrimental results for the community, the organization, and the careers of healthcare leaders are inevitable. But when related ethical implications are examined, the intent behind any proposed action can emerge. Actions that are motivated by greed or power, rather than mission or community need, quickly come to light, and the appearance of impropriety can be averted.

Decisions related to mergers, contracts, medical staff relations, human resources, budgeting, and program development all have ethical dimensions. Indeed, no management decision should be made without considering the ethical implications associated with it. How can a leader be most attuned to the ethical dimension, and how can she teach others to be more attuned than they are currently? As decisions are discussed, leaders throughout the management ranks must routinely examine the ethical implications of

Exhibit 3.1: The Interrelatedness of Ethics and Management

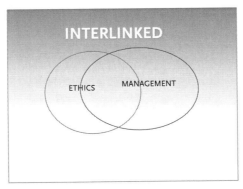

any action considered, just as they examine the financial and legal implications. Furthermore, ethical implications must be a part of any cost–benefit analysis and appear on the agenda of all management discussions.

Pitfall 2: Failing to Recognize That Management Decisions Directly Affect Clinical Care

Healthcare leaders recognize that their decisions lead to the financial success or failure of the organization and affect its position in the community. But how their decisions directly influence patient care is sometimes lost as attention is paid to the larger community. First, leaders are charged with adapting to the changes and addressing the threats of the external environment. Second, leaders are encouraged by their community and often by their board to be active and visible within the community, to advocate for population-based healthcare, and to establish the role and prominence of their organization in meeting population health needs. Attending to all these external issues may mask the direct impact of their management decisions on clinical care within their organizations.

> **"Don't create incentives** for unethical behavior. As we create goals for incentive compensation, think about what might backfire. When numbers are the goal, be specific about how numbers are to be attained.**"**
>
> **—Thomas C. Dolan,**
> **PhD, FACHE, CAE**

Another area in which management's direct impact on care may be obscured is operational decision making, Sometimes, hard decisions must be made related to staff reductions or closing patient care programs that are not financially viable. In addition to bottom-line considerations, attention must be paid to how such actions affect patient safety and healthcare needs. The patient care implications in these kinds of management decisions are clear, but they are not necessarily as clear in management decisions related to policy development or to medical staff credentialing, governing board appointments, human resources issues, or budgeting. Regardless, policies related to these issues and others directly affect clinical care, especially in the budgeting and resource allocation processes.

Healthcare leaders must always remember that the healthcare organization exists for the benefit of patients who place their lives in its care.

Pitfall 3: Failing to Integrate Ethics into Your Way of Conducting Business

Some healthcare executives believe that their ethics work is done once they have commanded that ethical standards of conduct or a values statement be developed, crafted into well-written language, and published in the annual report. Somehow, they must believe, the organization and all who are a part of it will become pillars of ethical behavior as a result of this action. But unless those values and standards are incorporated into the way of doing business day to day throughout the organization, they are useless. The real work begins as these values and standards are inculcated into the work life of every staff member, employee, and professional and are integrated

> **"Executive compensation is an issue today. Peter Drucker has** said that an executive's compensation should be no more than 25 times higher than the average employee. I have challenged CEOs to imagine themselves in a community town hall meeting where they are asked to justify their salary as compared to the salary of the most newly hired RN. Who has the greater impact on patient care?**"**
>
> **"Society's emphasis on wealth and worldly goods has an** influence on ethical behavior. How we craft our incentive programs can impact behavior. Executives on quarterly incentive programs are unlikely to take on initiatives that require a few years to demonstrate success.**"**
>
> **—Patrick G. Hays, FACHE**

into every activity from the boardroom to housekeeping. Values must be "discussed at every opportunity, constantly reinforced and consistently reflected in the actions of management at all levels" (George 2003, 72).

Pitfall 4: Failing to Understand That Just Because an Action Is Legal Does Not Mean It Is Ethical

George (2003) also cites a quote by a Harvard classmate of Enron CEO Jeff Skilling noting that Skilling would argue in class "that the role of the business leader was to take advantage of loopholes in regulations and push beyond the laws wherever he could to make money . . . it was the job of the regulators to try and catch him." Far too many leaders on Wall Street and beyond have adopted this philosophy, and society has suffered for it. In 2003, in the wake of the many incidents of corporate misconduct, Harvard Business School replaced its three-week ethics module with a new, required, semester-long ethics course that includes an Enron Corporation case study (Weisman 2003).

Pushing legal boundaries does not build leadership character. In his book *Authentic Leadership*,

George (2003, 16) shares a philosophy espoused by the late US Representative Amory Houghton (R-NY) related to legality versus ethics. He believed we are all surrounded by concentric circles. The outer circle is made up of the laws, regulations, and ethical standards with which the organization must comply. The inner circle is made up of the personal core values of the individual leader. Houghton advised leaders to never act in a manner that reaches beyond the inner circle of core values even though the action may be deemed legal. Certainly, healthcare leaders must heed the constraints of the laws and seek the legal opinions and advice of attorneys, but they must also recognize that management decisions require much more consideration than simply, "Is it legal?" The role of the attorney is to advise—it is the healthcare leader who must decide. Morally sound management decision making considers all dimensions of the process, including ethical implications and impact on numerous constituencies and stakeholders.

Pitfall 5: Believing You Are Above the Laws and Rules of "Ordinary Men"

Collins' (2001) research for his book *Good to Great* found that great companies consistently were headed by leaders with "a combination of humility and professional will." Hesselbein and Shrader (2008, 35) concur: "Cultures around the world that have endured for hundreds and thousands of years invariably come to value humility as an attribute of real leadership." Without humility, we cannot see our biases or prejudices and how they influence our views of society. Too often, those at the top of successful organizations come to believe that success occurs because of them and their leadership, and they develop a sense of entitlement to personal rewards. In a society where

> **"ACHE has Integrity as one of its Standards of Excellence for Staff. You either meet that standard or not."**
>
> —Thomas C. Dolan, PhD, FACHE, CAE

wealth is equated with success, wealth may become the goal, and personal gain becomes more important than organizational success. In the corporate world, this sense of entitlement may be manifested in tax avoidance through offshore headquarters, the shutdown of worthwhile projects that do not pay off immediately, staff reductions to increase the bottom line, or manipulation of financial figures to increase executive bonuses (George 2003, 4). Human nature dictates that "the more successful we are, the more tempted we are to take short-cuts to keep it going" to prove that we are a legitimate success (George 2003, 17).

> **"I attend** new-employee orientation, give out my e-mail address, and tell the employees to let me know if they have concerns about whether we are meeting our [ethical] standards.**"**
>
> **—Nancy M. Schlichting**

Great leaders sometimes possess major character flaws. Zenger and Folkman (2002, 57) call this trait "the Clinton phenomenon." Like President Bill Clinton, they argue, such leaders may not lose their job or go to jail, but they cause irreparable damage to their reputations and their relationships nonetheless. Trust and confidence in these leaders may never be restored. Healthcare leaders are not exempt from temptation. Prominent, successful leaders have been caught up in humiliating, unethical, and sometimes illegal acts. Their misdeeds tend to focus on financial or sexual transgressions as a result of escalating executive arrogance.

Healthcare leaders must set high standards and practice the standards they expect of employees. They cannot operate by one set of rules and expect their employees to function under a different, higher set of standards.

Pitfall 6: Rushing to Judgment

Ask any healthcare leader what is his most precious resource. Chances are, he will answer "time." Healthcare is a beleaguered industry, blamed for rising healthcare costs, assailed for contributing to the national deficit, and idling at the center of the national health-care reform mandate demanding value for money. Clearly healthcare leaders feel pressed for time.

While advances in technology allow leaders to save time per-forming some tasks, technology may also have become the enemy of thoughtful reflection and creativity. David Brooks (2007) says we pay a cost for our "wireless life," in which we are constantly bombarded with information and data and are expected to react, not reflect.

Furthermore, aspiring healthcare leaders may mistakenly believe that the ability to make rapid, independent decisions is the mark of a high-performing leader, and they may fear that failure to do so will be interpreted as a failure in leadership. In reality, a healthcare manager is confronted with ethical dilemmas on a daily basis. Most of the time, unconsciously, the manager makes the right decision. Most individuals involved in healthcare are decent, moral people who are attracted to the healthcare field because they wish to contribute valuable work to society. Inevitably, however, errors in judgment, detrimental decisions, and unintentional mis-takes are made. Mistakes are often the result of hurried decisions made without the benefit of the thoughtful reflection and the con-sultation of others. On a practical level, too little time, too little thought, and too little dialogue are routinely devoted to exploring the ethical issues imbedded in management decisions.

The key to ethical decision making is an awareness of the necessity to ask thoughtful questions and take the time to formu-late ethically sound answers. Successful healthcare leaders refuse to rush to judgment in order to avoid making hasty decisions that may not account for the ethical implications.

Pitfall 7: Believing That When Everyone Else Does It, You Can Do It, Too

As we have noted, healthcare is a microcosm of society, and social observers such as Joanne Lipman (2011) warn that the Judeo-

Christian values on which the United States was founded are insidiously being replaced with moral relativism, whereby the standards of right and wrong are mere products of time and culture and morality is nothing more than a neutral concept. In healthcare, the encroaching moral relativism may be playing out through the economic downturn and recent new challenges facing healthcare. Is the current healthcare environment making it more difficult for executives to maintain ethical standards of conduct? In other words, if everyone in society seems to be bending the rules, doesn't that mean that it's OK for us to do so? If we don't bend the rules like everyone else, will we remain competitive? Experienced healthcare leaders know that bending the rules for short-term gains may have long-term negative consequences. Inevitably, questionable legal or ethical behavior will come to light and any competitive gain will be lost.

> **The greatest deterrent to unethical behavior is education as to** what's ethical and what's not. Using scenarios is the best way to do this. Today's university programs are not teaching this. These are our future leaders, and we need to be giving them a better understanding of what constitutes ethical behavior. Unfortunately, we all think we are ethical.
>
> —**Donald C. Wegmiller,** FACHE

BUILDING AN ETHICAL INFRASTRUCTURE

To leave a lasting and positive legacy, healthcare executives are encouraged to build an ethical infrastructure to inoculate their careers from these seven pitfalls to ethical decision making. When leaders see ethics as "a practical tool used to enhance decision making and shape organizational practices and policies" (Freund 2010), they will create an ethical culture in their organizations that makes ethics the only acceptable way of doing business, thereby increasing their chances of success.

Steps to creating a culture that promotes and supports ethical conduct may include the following:

1. Establish ethical standards and expectations.
   - Make it known to all stakeholders, constituencies, and partners and to the public that your organization "lives" its ethical standards and expects nothing less of those it works with to deliver healthcare.
   - Hire ethical people. Make sure the interview process determines to the extent possible that candidates share the organization's values. Pose scenarios of ethical dilemmas to assess candidates' values.
   - Cultivate a relationship with a trusted colleague within or outside your organization who can serve as a candid and honest confidant regarding the appearance of your conduct. Use this trusted source to discuss ethical dilemmas and potential actions, in both the personal and professional arenas.

2. Establish a code of ethical conduct.
   - Develop a code of ethical conduct with the governing board, professional and nonprofessional staff, and bargaining unit representatives if the organization is unionized, making certain that all are invested in its development and

> **"The greatest deterrent is the consistent and absolute intolerance** of unethical behavior. A policy of zero tolerance means swift action is taken when it occurs, regardless of organizational status. Prerequisites include:
> - A comprehensive and unambiguous code of conduct that is well disseminated and understood.
> - No disconnect between the rhetoric and reality of organizational values.
> - Behavior of all organizational leaders and staff members that is always beyond reproach."
>
> **—Paul B. Hofmann,** DrPH, FACHE

promotion. For an example of an organizational code of ethical conduct, see Appendix A, "American College of Healthcare Executives (ACHE) *Code of Ethics*."

- Introduce and distribute the code throughout the organization. Leaders must have a visible role in this effort so that the importance of the code of conduct is known to all.
- Rethink the code of conduct periodically to ensure that it is current with ethical demands.

> **"The biggest** deterrent to unethical behavior is the upbringing that employees bring to the organization. Since an ethical background cannot be taken for granted, in-service education is a critical key to ethical conduct."
>
> **—Thomas C. Dolan,**
> **PhD, FACHE, CAE**

3. Role model ethical standards.
   - Leaders must exemplify ethical standards of behavior on a personal and professional level and challenge staff and employees to do the same, especially those in visible leadership positions.
   - Leaders must be vigilant in monitoring their conduct to ensure that they are not guilty of misdeeds that make a mockery of the organization's ethical position.
   - Leaders should periodically complete an ethics self-assessment, such as that published by ACHE (see Appendix I), to discover any opportunities for further reflection regarding their ethical leadership and actions.

> **"Integrity must be modeled at the very top of the organization** with the board and with the executive office. Transparency needs to be ever present. Special attention needs to be placed on conflict-of-interest policies and enforcement at the board level. Executive privilege requires review, and policies need to address personal expenses. Ground rules for acceptable entertainment and gifts and firm guidelines for relationships between purchasing agents and suppliers will do much to deter unethical behaviors."
>
> **—John G. King, LFACHE**

4. Establish an ethics committee.
   - The ethics committee should include representation from a wide range of disciplines, such as physicians, theologians, nurses, patient advocates, attorneys, ethicists, researchers, senior management, and the community. Some healthcare organizations ask former patients or their family members to serve on the committee.
   - The ethics committee must be charged with the authority to oversee both clinical and business ethics issues.
   - The ethics committee must have a prominent role in the organization and, while advisory in nature, must speak with expert authority.
   - Ethics committee members must be appropriately trained in ethical decision making and well versed in organizational policy and standards of care within the community.
   - The referral process and the role and responsibility of the ethics committee must be made known throughout the organization.

5. Develop ethics training and education.
   - Require ethics training and education in staff development throughout the organization, with programming appropriate to all staff levels.
   - Include ethics training in all new-employee orientations.
   - Use real-world case studies in education sessions. This approach is highly effective in integrating ethical standards as a way of thinking in the organization (George 2003, 132).
   - Establish forums in which employees can talk about values and find common ground and in which values can be publicly affirmed.

6. Ensure compliance with ethical standards.
   - Establish systems that ensure compliance, enforcement, punishment for improper actions, and rewards for ethical conduct.

- Establish an anonymous hotline for anyone who wishes to provide information regarding potential ethical breaches.
- Create the position of ethics officer or compliance officer, with education, consultation, and oversight responsibilities.

7. Create an ethical environment for employees.

> **"Ethical behavior should be** rewarded. What gets measured gets managed; what gets rewarded gets done."
>
> **—Thomas C. Dolan,** PhD, FACHE, CAE

  - Be aware that leadership's ethical responsibilities to the people they work with and manage are just as important as their responsibilities to patients, clients, and others served.
  - Create a work environment free from harassment, discrimination, or any pressures to perform or ignore illegal or unethical acts.
  - Establish fair and equitable practices regarding recruitment, hiring, performance evaluation, and firing. The firing of an employee should be conducted with honesty, clear explanation, fairness, and respect and should enable the employee to retain as much dignity and self-respect as possible.
  - Establish performance evaluations that reward ethical conduct and correct unethical conduct.

> **"It is critical that** there be a safe haven for people to come forward with ethical concerns. Healthcare leaders must create this safe environment so that employees do not fear retaliation for any concerns expressed."
>
> **—John G. King,** LFACHE

> **"'Doing the right thing' gets more** complex and challenging the higher you reach in the organization and the longer you have been in your career. This is especially true at the CEO level. Caution to avoid conflict of interest must be routinely exercised because of the many personal and professional relationships that develop over the years."
>
> **—David J. Fine,** FACHE

- Institute ethical workforce reduction policies. Staff retraining or reassignment, severance policies, outplacement, counseling, and clear and honest communication are important factors to consider in this process.
- Address impairment in the workplace. Widespread professional staff and employee education must include signs, symptoms, and dangers of impairment to the impaired and to others. Patient safety must be of paramount concern.
- Establish reporting mechanisms, counseling, and treatment options for impairment.
- Avoid any appearance of personal impairment.
- Take a leadership role in creating an ethical culture. Do not delegate these responsibilities to the human resources department and assume that your time is better spent focusing on the financial viability or the competitive advantage of the organization. Recognize that by taking a leadership role in creating an ethical culture for employees, you are improving the organization's financial and competitive position.

8. Integrate a patient's bill of rights into operations.
   - Create a living patient's bill of rights and educate employees, patients, and families about its existence and content.
   - Establish customer service or patient advocacy programs as dictated by the needs of the population served.

9. Adopt a framework for ethical decision making.
   - Add ethical implications to the agenda when decisions are being made at the board, management, and program levels.
   - Make values-based decisions by naming, clarifying, and weighing the values at stake in deciding the issue, make appropriate decisions on the basis of these values, and communicate the decisions and the reasoning behind them accurately and thoroughly (Perry 2001, 22) (see Exhibit 3.2).

Exhibit 3.2: Decision-Making Ellipse

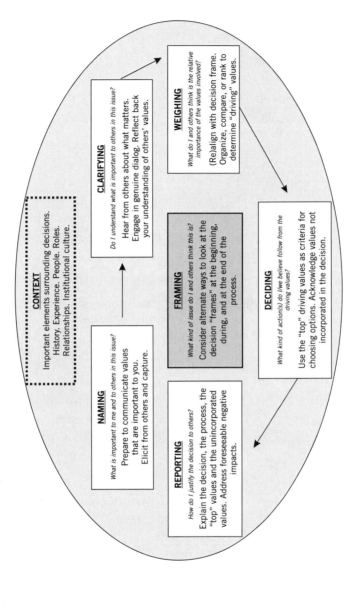

CONTEXT
Important elements surrounding decisions. History. Experience. People. Roles. Relationships. Institutional culture.

NAMING
What is important to me and to others in this issue?
Prepare to communicate values that are important to you.
Elicit from others and capture.

CLARIFYING
Do I understand what is important to others in this issue?
Hear from others about what matters. Engage in genuine dialog. Reflect back your understanding of others' values.

WEIGHING
What do I and others think is the relative importance of the values involved?
(Re)align with decision frame. Organize, compare, or rank to determine "driving" values.

FRAMING
What kind of issue do I and others think this is?
Consider alternate ways to look at the decision "frames" at the beginning, during, and at the end of the process.

REPORTING
How do I justify the decision to others?
Explain the decision, the process, the "top" values and the unincorporated values. Address foreseeable negative impacts.

DECIDING
What kind of action(s) do I/we believe follow from the driving values?
Use the "top" driving values as criteria for choosing options. Acknowledge values not incorporated in the decision.

Source: Copyright 2000. Mark Bennett and Joan McIver Gibson. Permission granted to copy and use with attribution.

- Make certain that ethical decisions adhere to the mission, vision, ethical standards, and values of the organization.

10. Invite colleagues to continually review and enhance your ethical culture.
    - Ensure that ethical standards are current with ethical demands and that practices are consistent and in keeping with standards.
    - Make sure that staff education is up to date and widely disseminated.

THE BUSINESS CASE FOR ETHICS

Character is not a secondary attribute of leadership; it is the driver that propels a career of impact. Legacy leaders know that ethics is not an ethereal discipline embraced only by theologians and philosophers. Ethics plays an essential role in the intricate set of actions taken in making morally sound management decisions that lead to personal and organizational success.

Physicians and employees in healthcare are hungry to work with leaders who inspire and challenge them to achieve high levels of ethical performance. Staff and employees are only willing to follow leaders who demonstrate a strong character and high integrity and are worthy of their loyalty and commitment. The ability to inspire and motivate others is strongly linked to a leader's perceived level of integrity (Zenger and Folkman 2002, 79).

Strength of character requires discipline and progressive reinforcement, and leaders who wish to create a career of impact are consciously aware of this need. They are unfailing in their efforts to build an ethical culture and a legacy of character. Throughout their careers, these leaders are intentional about setting high standards and leading by example. Those who do will find that an enhanced public image of the organization will attract competent, ethical staff and physicians; patients who seek trustworthy care;

and insurers that want to do business with a reputable organization. As the Association of Academic Health Centers maintains, "The essence of a profession is that its members commit themselves to a set of standards higher than the morals of the marketplace."

THREE KEY ACTIONS TO HARDWIRE INTEGRITY AND CHARACTER INTO YOUR LEGACY ROAD MAP

Action 1: Complete the ACHE "Ethics Self-Assessment" (see Appendix I or visit www.ache.org) and strengthen identified areas with additional reading and education. Require direct reports to do the same.

Action 2: Make a conscious effort to role model values and stress the importance of matching actions with values. Participate in case-based ethics education, made available to all levels of employees, that features specific and reflective real-world work situations or dilemmas. Encourage open discussion among staff.

Action 3: Routinely include ethical implications on the agenda when management actions are being considered and are a part of any cost–benefit analysis.

CHAPTER 4

Visioning: The Long View

A VISION IS a clear description of a desired future state of being, whether applied to organizations or individuals. Healthcare leaders who strive for a career of impact must cultivate a desired vision that defines how both their organization and their career will look and behave in the future.

Visioning is the art and science of developing and then bringing into sharp focus a bold view of how reality will look and behave at a specified time in the future, say, summer 2020. When leaders invite stakeholders to help develop, to embrace, and to work intentionally toward achieving the organization's vision, colleagues and staff are not only engaged with and share ownership of that vision but also more likely to work harder to achieve it.

And so it is with one's personal vision. The leader who adopts an intentional process to achieve clarity and boldness of vision for a career of impact improves the probability that she will experience such a career. Her chances are even higher if she includes respected mentors, colleagues, or her spouse in candid conversations about the vision.

DISCIPLINED DOING: MAP YOUR ACTIONS

Interview after interview with the healthcare leaders featured in this book suggested that legacies are not the result of wishful thinking.

They are intentional and inspirational. They are the result of disciplined doing.

Looking back on their active and successful careers, top healthcare leaders assert that the life you lead can benefit from a clearly marked, and periodically updated, legacy road map. They recommend that, rather than drifting through life, you establish your career journey by using what Schwartz (1991) calls "the long view" to build a bold vision of your career 10 to 20 years from now. If you have not done so already, draft your preferred obituary (see Action 3 at the end of Chapter 1) today to influence your approach to your work for tomorrow. But, as we advise earlier, do not just put your head in the clouds; keep your feet on the ground as well. Think of your daily commitment to disciplined doing as plotting the landmarks for your legacy road map.

Despite observations from our interviewed executives about their need to be concerned about the future, the most important leadership actions are those you take today. Kouzes and Posner (2006, 180) note that "You never know when that critical moment might come. What you do know is that you can make a difference. You can leave this world better than you found it." Just as we lead our lives daily, we leave our legacy daily, and that understanding is key to disciplined doing. In addition to guiding you to your desired future state, a legacy road map allows you to imagine alternate scenarios for your career path and destination. Permit yourself to do a bit of dreaming as you draft these scenarios. Schwartz (1991, 4) comments that scenarios are "a set of organized ways for us to dream effectively about our own future. They resemble a set of stories, either written out or often spoken. However, these stories are built around carefully constructed 'plots' that make the significant elements of the world scene stand out boldly." Effective healthcare leaders

> **"Great leaders have** great vision. I have tried to focus an important dimension of my vision and leadership to embrace evidence-based medicine and enhanced quality."
>
> —Gail L. Warden, LFACHE

continuously frame and reframe alternate scenarios for their organizations as well as for their careers. It is within these scenarios that legacy leaders craft road maps to explore the best path to the envisioned future.

As you design your legacy road map to reflect your preferred career vision scenarios, follow this five-step process:

1. Draft two headlines to your obituary: one that captures what you will have achieved in your professional career and one that summarizes inspiring comments from the eulogy given by a valued family member or friend.
2. Conduct two candid "gap analyses": one that assesses the differences between the aspirational, professional, and personal headlines and one that assesses the gap between your current performance in each of these headlined arenas and your desired position. Be honest and probing.
3. Reflect on two to three of the most important factors that could frustrate, and two to three factors that could facilitate, your successful achievement of the legacy attributes in the two gap analyses. Enter your answers in the matrix shown below.

	Professional legacy gap	Personal legacy gap
Factors likely to frustrate		
Factors likely to facilitate		

4. Brainstorm with trusted mentors and family members the handful of actions you should take to avoid the frustration factors (taboos) and to embrace the facilitation factors (dos).
5. Commit to taking the first steps of your journey to implement these actions and to periodically revisit and refine your action plans.

Kouzes and Posner (2006, 179) conclude that while looking forward may be the quality that differentiates leaders from other credible people, the future does not belong to leaders alone. Leaders are custodians of the desired future, and their constituents and followers are its occupants. Your followers must participate in shaping their roles in your legacy. Therefore, effective leaders turn their followers into leaders, and they are willing to become followers (Atchison 2004). In today's complex health systems, in which staffs are participating in scores of process improvement teams, frontline workers will lead tasks while senior managers play a supportive follower role. In other words, situations will occasionally require situational leaders rather than titled leaders.

Mapping your actions through disciplined doing includes pinpointing those circumstances in which your leadership is enhanced by being a follower.

Visioning Is Not Enough: Execution Matters

Personifying your career plan through your actions requires successful execution and skillful change management. Leading change to achieve success in the long term is a more subtle approach than "creating a burning platform" to overcome the fear of change. Steve Crom (2012) describes five myths about change that legacy leaders must dispel.

Myth 1: Change is easier when you are in a crisis.

Myth 2: Fundamental change has to be revolutionary change.

Myth 3: Before we change, we have to be clear about our destination.

Myth 4: Change management is done by professional change agents.

Myth 5: Most people resist change because they are afraid.

He proposes the following formula to help leaders overcome institutional resistance to needed change:

$$Improvement = (A + B + C) > X,$$

where A = dissatisfaction with the current condition, B = clarity about the new condition, C = the way to get to the new condition, and X = the cost of change in terms of both money and psychological or social factors (adapted from Crom 2012).

Legacy leaders must map a path for themselves and their teams that optimizes the management of these variables for project, organization, and career improvement. Success is more likely to occur if leaders can consider each variable's contribution to motivate themselves as well as others toward a promising future.

CAREER ENVISIONING

The Center for Creative Leadership has long championed fresh approaches to developing leaders and increasing their effectiveness. Its recent exploration of innovative thinking, highlighted in the six steps that follow, can be applied to a healthcare leader who is engaging in strategic visioning for a career of impact (Horth and Buchner 2009).

1. *Paying attention.* Literally look and listen from a new perspective. Read autobiographies of leaders you admire. Talk with respected healthcare leaders who are leaving legacies you admire.
2. *Personalizing.* Understand your customer's or patient's experience in a deep, personal way.
3. *Exploring imaging.* Pictures, stories, impressions, and metaphors are powerful tools for describing situations, constructing ideas, and communicating effectively. Consider which images best capture your dreams for your career over the next 20 years.

4. *Seriously playing.* Visioning and innovation require bending some rules, branching out, and having some fun. Improvisation, experimentation, levity, and rapid prototyping work may feel like play, but the results are serious business.
5. *Practicing collaborative inquiry.* Confer with the person with whom you can most comfortably discuss your career fears and aspirations. In addition, network with leaders in other industries to converse about career plans.
6. *Crafting.* Through abductive reasoning, we can make intuitive connections among seemingly unrelated information and begin to shape order out of what may seem to be a chaotic career path.

Another aid in career envisioning is literature from other disciplines and industries. Consider which sources to include to stimulate your thinking about servant leadership, careers of influence, and personal growth.

Career Visions Benefit from Succession Planning

A few years ago, we invited Marshall Goldsmith, one of the most widely cited executive coaches in North America, to our Cambridge, England, International Health Leadership Program. The conversation we had about his work with leaders in other industries was provocative. He shared the idea that succession planning equates to legacy planning. Great leaders develop their own succession plan not only to ensure leadership continuity for their organization but also to fully establish and solidify their career road map. They also guide their direct reports in developing succession plans and road maps so they, too, may achieve careers of impact.

Our work across many health systems shows a discouraging lack of succession planning and leadership development. Boards, physicians, staff, and donors become frustrated and distracted from mission-critical work in the face of unplanned executive departures. The US health sector lags other service industries in making the investment in succession planning and leadership pipeline development.

Ram Charan (2008b, 21) concludes that most leadership development processes and training programs do not enable executives to achieve personal or organization success, no matter how much money we spend on them, because they are built on serious shortcomings in understanding about leadership and its development, including the following:

- Failing to recognize that only a few people have the potential to run a major organization and that these people must be spotted early to spare them the torture of having to prove themselves on every rung in a ten-step vertical ladder.
- Failing to make the identification and development of future leaders an explicit part of every executive's job, to provide the tools to do it, and to reward those who do it well. Healthcare organizations track a leader's ability to produce numbers, but not her ability to produce other leaders; you must reverse this trend to build a career of impact.
- Relegating the early identification and development of high-potential successors to lower-level leaders who are ill prepared for the task.
- Using perfunctory and bureaucratic performance reviews as a coaching and career-planning device.
- Applying the same expectations and job rotations to all leaders, rather than customizing them to an individual's talents and development needs.
- Spreading leadership development resources across too many leaders in hopes that strong candidates will emerge.
- Using classroom education as a substitute for real-world challenges.

When reflecting on the succession planning and career development of legacy leaders, Goldsmith (2009, 17) observes that "Almost all of the leaders who I have met assure me that *they* will be different. They confidently assert that *they* will have no problems letting go. You are probably delusional enough to believe that *you* too will be different. Take my word for it, while your desire for uniqueness may be theoretically possible, it is statistically unlikely" (emphasis in original). Legacy leaders, on the other hand, drive themselves and their colleagues in an intentional manner to achieve long-view visions of their career by establishing a formal succession plan. These succession plans provide not only personal stability and continuity but also continuity and stability for your organization.

The advisers at Integrated Healthcare Strategies (www.ihstrat egies.com) work with health system executives and boards to bolster organizational performance by supporting leadership continuity when executives retire or relocate. Key questions to shape the succession plan are the following (IHS n.d.):

- Has the board reached consensus with the executive team about the competencies needed in the ideal senior leadership group of the future?
- Has the board acknowledged the disruption to the organization resulting from unplanned executive departures?
- Has a clear process for executive transition been planned to optimize stability for the organization, its senior leadership team, and the departing executive(s)?
- How will the ideal map of competencies needed in the leadership team of the future be developed on an ongoing basis to ensure organizational continuity, focus on results, and drive toward the mission and vision of the enterprise?
- How should the organization invest in a culture that nurtures ongoing leadership development, mentoring, and coaching for enhanced stability and continuity of leadership in turbulent times?

Once they have answered these questions, health system boards and CEOs should develop the following processes to shore up their succession planning (IHS n.d.):

- Targeted training and development for the best and brightest in the organization to move into career pathways that simultaneously grow their competencies and strengthen the organization's prospects for success
- The parameters and scope of a sound mentoring program in which personal and professional growth occur for both mentor and mentee
- Identification of people who are best suited to be mentors to achieve the vision, and their training needs
- Identification of the best protégé candidates and the pairings that make the most sense to maximize that relationship

Though the benefits of this process may not be quantified in one or two quarters or even in a year, the leaders will know that their efforts are geared toward the long-term success and vitality of their organizations. They will know that through a holistic succession and development plan, they are building a leadership legacy that will outlive them.

Followers Earned

Your career vision must explicitly include attention to followers. These followers have to be earned through engagement and empowerment.

Effective leaders recognize that however smart they are, they are not smarter than everyone else combined. They appreciate that not only do the same rules apply to them, perhaps they apply even more because leaders' behavior is seen as setting the standard for others. Legacy leaders are vigilant in recognizing their mistakes and admitting to them before they are printed in the press or disclosed in another public forum. They cannot lose sight of the fact that no matter how important their own contributions are, they could not have advanced their career without the help and hard work of many other people (Kouzes and Posner 2006, 159, 160).

Atchison (2004) suggests three attributes that leaders who envision a career of impact should engender in their staff to ensure a strong cultural environment that includes inspired followers:

1. Followers need to find *meaning* in their work.
2. Followers need to be *respected*.
3. Followers need a *sense of control*.

A well-conceived legacy road map enables you to build organization and team cultures in which you earn followers by maintaining a strong sense of meaning, respect, and control. When you communicate a clear vision for the organization and your followers that is aligned with your legacy road map, you bring them closer to fulfilling that vision.

THREE KEY ACTIONS TO HARDWIRE VISIONING INTO YOUR LEGACY ROAD MAP

Action 1: Use self-reflection and scenario-based strategic thinking to scan the future and clearly define the vision you have for your career of impact. Explore how your vision interacts with the vision forged for your organization.

Action 2: Move beyond words that express your career vision, and embrace behaviors and actions that show others your passion and initiatives to achieve the vision, with and for the followers whom you earn.

Action 3: Commit to be more disciplined in your development of succession plans for your direct reports.

CHAPTER 5

Mentoring and Leadership Development

OUR WORK WITH leaders of all ages and demographic profiles, in diverse types of health-sector organizations, reinforces our belief in the importance of mentoring to support not only a career of impact but also the long-term success and vitality of the healthcare organization. Healthcare leaders know that mentoring matters but may not know how to develop and implement a mentorship program. Our interviews with 21 successful healthcare leaders offer several useful insights, including the observation that their career advancement and sense of purpose were instilled through early guidance provided by a respected mentor.

As Sandstrom and Smith (2008, 21) found, legacy leadership is about building people, not building things. The healthcare leaders interviewed for this book indicated they often exhibited the value of cultivating their mentoring effectiveness through intentional leadership team development—by allocating some of their time to and sharing relevant career experiences with their direct reports. They communicated their appreciation for the power of mentoring as well as an expectation that those whom they mentor will mentor others in turn. Mentoring initiatives set a tone from the top that leverages the legacy leader's investment manyfold.

If you are a healthcare leader—of a hospital, a department, a clinic, or any group of individuals—you will leave a leadership legacy in direct proportion to your effectiveness as a mentor. Your legacy will not be a record of how you behaved or a report card of your healthcare organization's performance (although that is how it might be summed up by the press). Instead, as mentioned earlier, your legacy will be revealed in how your colleagues, employees, and others think and behave as a result of the time they spent working with you (Galford and Maruca 2006, 3–4).

Mentoring is not easy. Many healthcare organizations have launched mentoring programs only to see them hampered by a lack of clear direction or by poor pairings of unsuitable, untrained mentors with incompatible protégés. The administration of these initiatives is often delegated to the human resources department, which lacks the leadership investment and appropriate authority to implement an effective mentoring program. Instead, mentoring should begin with the board and CEO; legacies rise and fall in relation to how supportive the mentoring culture is.

> **"My family inspired a hunger to gather and apply knowledge, and** be prepared for hard work. My curiosity and willingness to work hard moved me through a series of studies and leadership positions in academic medicine.
> I think great leaders act as 'accelerators' to the work and talents of those around them. My grandfather would say . . . 'If you have a gift and you don't use it, no confessor on earth can absolve you!'**"**
> **—Patricia Gabow, MD**

DEVELOPING OTHERS MATTERS

How do great leaders become good mentors? Most of our interviews suggest that mentors provide exceptional learning experiences for their mentees. These learning experiences not only expand their mentee's awareness, insights, and perspectives but also enrich the organization's capacity for enhanced performance and pride by instituting a culture of development.

A culture of development is more likely to emerge when mentoring is a component of the expected way of thinking and working throughout the organization. In such an environment, creating opportunities for growth and peak performance becomes the norm when people in middle management and on the front lines are able to observe how the senior leaders behave in their relationships and witness their intentional investment of time and effort to reach out and develop others around them.

Legacy leaders, therefore, intentionally influence and develop other leaders. Amid the complexity of today's multigenerational healthcare workforce, they must be prepared to build a multigenerational culture. The old "command and control" style of leadership is no longer effective. Smart workers expect more and different competencies from their leaders, and they require more and better reasons to excel than merely producing profit for someone else. Employees expect leaders to be interested in them, not just the bottom line. Long-term corporate loyalty is outdated, with employees holding more positions and making more career changes during their working lives than ever before.

> **"I try to have five principles guide my work: collaboration,** communication, trust, integrity, respect. We should try to select, promote, and develop people who we believe have the best potential to embrace and master these five key qualities.
>
> Job one should be 'leaders developing leaders,' not just leaders who can eventually take our place tomorrow, but leaders whom we will enjoy working with today.**"**
>
> **—Mark R. Tolosky, JD, FACHE**

> **"Mentoring is an important attribute of great leaders. I was** mentored by Don Carver, and I strive to be a good mentor. A related core value should be: 'It all starts with people; picking the right people is one of a leader's most important responsibilities.'**"**
>
> **—Stanley R. Nelson, LFACHE**

Effective legacy planning asks how best to earn followers among a multigenerational workforce and how to develop leaders throughout that workforce. Leadership development strategies and organizational infrastructure to support these generations become essential challenges to and targets for your legacy road map. But only a few hospitals and healthcare systems have begun to establish an internal development pipeline culture or a "university" to accommodate the multigenerational workforce. Organizations need to build internal resources and systems that enable the generation of future leaders and assist with the continuous development of staff.

Charan (2008a, 1) asserts that few organizations are well prepared for such internal leadership development. He rightly reminds us that the first law of holes—when you're in one, stop digging—tells us what to do: Abandon our traditional leadership development practices; they are not working. Charan notes, "Tinkering and fine-tuning won't solve the fundamental problem. It's time for a completely new approach to finding and developing the kinds of leaders businesses need. Companies need to reinvent their leadership development processes and for individual leaders to guide their own careers."

Kouzes and Posner's (2006) work with hundreds of organizations concludes that this lack of preparation is more a function of flaws in the leader's attitude than a lack of effective leadership

> **❝Successful leaders work with and learn from strong board leaders.** Bob Hanberg, of Boise Cascade, is. Bob encouraged a disciplined approach to community service.
>
> Tom Atchison reminds us that managers are like farmers; we don't grow crops, we create an environment in which crops can grow.
>
> Great leaders leave a legacy by creating an environment in which others can grow.❞
>
> **—Ed Dahlberg, LFACHE**

development programs. Kirk Hanson, university professor and executive director of the Markkula Center for Applied Ethics at Santa Clara University, says leaders must avoid the following common traps (cited in Kouzes and Posner 2006):

- Believe they know it all
- Believe they are in charge
- Believe the rules don't apply to them
- Believe they will never fail
- Believe they did it all by themselves
- Believe they are better than the "little people"
- Believe they *are* the organization
- Believe they can focus everything on the job

> **"Who shaped my career?**
> Great mentors: Walter McNerney; Jim Campbell, MD, at Rush; and Alex McMahon of the American Hospital Association.
>   A mentoring role is key, and I have tried especially to be a champion to mentor and promote women into healthcare leadership roles.**"**
>   —**Gail L. Warden**, LFACHE

Legacy leaders can forge and follow a legacy road map that helps them avoid these pitfalls.

WHAT MAKES A GOOD MENTOR?

Our work with health system leaders in more than 30 countries suggests many answers to the question, What makes a good mentor? The following responses are a sampling:

- One who cares about the mentee
- One who knows he grows as he shares insights with his mentees
- One who demonstrates active listening
- One who recognizes he does not have all the answers
- One who is willing to take the time to be an active mentor

Mentoring does not require special skills, but mentors should be good role models. Great mentors exhibit the behaviors and style they hope to see in their mentees. Two sets of mentoring guidelines—one developed by Blue Sky Coaching in Australia (www.blueskycoaching.com.au) and one created by the Connecticut Mentoring Partnership—can help healthcare leaders develop their competencies as mentors.

To be more intentional in your approach to mentoring, we encourage you to embrace the 12 traits shown in Exhibit 5.1. Variations on the points outlined in Exhibit 5.1 are offered in Exhibit 5.2.

> **"My career in healthcare was shaped by an early interest in being** a physician. My career path quickly shifted to management and the fun of getting work done with and through others. I see effective leadership in those [who] earn followers; those who always look for the big-picture view; [those who] support the development of young managers; and, very importantly, [those who are] clear what you want to stand for—being a leader is a privilege; you can influence others."
>
> **—Nancy M. Schlichting**

> **"As chief resident and then later as a physician executive, I found** a growing curiosity in the value of leveraging an individual's talent through the work of groups and teams.
>
> Ron Anderson, MD, CEO of Parkland, became a mentor [who] opened additional doors of opportunity to help grow medical practice and participate in strategic thinking and business planning. Physician leaders have an opportunity to help organizations thrive by serving as an effective 'translator' among business and clinical colleagues. We too often talk past or over each other, and not communicate clearly enough about what we are trying to accomplish, and how we think the process needs to work to accomplish it."
>
> **—Samuel L. Ross, MD**

Exhibit 5.1: Mentor Competencies

1. Mentors listen.

   They maintain eye contact and give mentees their full attention.

2. Mentors guide.

   Mentors are there to help their mentees find life direction, never to push them.

3. Mentors are practical.

   They give insights about keeping on task and setting goals and priorities.

4. Mentors educate.

   Mentors educate about life and their own careers.

5. Mentors provide insight.

   Mentors use their personal experience to help their mentees avoid mistakes and learn from good decisions.

6. Mentors are accessible.

   Mentors are available as a resource and a sounding board.

7. Mentors criticize constructively.

   When necessary, mentors point out areas that need improvement, always focusing on the mentee's behavior, never his/her character.

8. Mentors are supportive.

   No matter how painful the mentee's experience, mentors continue to encourage them to learn and improve.

9. Mentors are specific.

   Mentors give specific advice on what was done well or could be corrected, what was achieved and the benefits of various actions.

10. Mentors care.

    Mentors care about their mentees' progress in school and career planning, as well as their personal development.

11. Mentors succeed.

    Mentors not only are successful themselves, but they also foster success in others.

12. Mentors are admirable.

    Mentors are usually well respected in their organizations and in the community.

Source: Connecticut Mentoring Partnership and Business and Legal Reports (1999). Used with permission from the Connecticut Mentoring Partnership and the Business and Legal Reports, Inc.

Exhibit 5.2: Mentoring Milestones

1. **Be credible**
    The best mentors . . . have been people that have credibility in, and have personally achieved [organizational] success. . . . For this reason, most people will seek the guidance of different mentors to help them develop specific skills or qualities, or to help them reach important decisions. Being credible doesn't mean that you need to have all the answers. The best answers for your mentee will come from their own thinking, with the help of your wisdom to support them.

2. **Be a positive role model**
    Good mentors are respected by their mentees. A mentee can learn a lot from their mentor simply by watching how their mentor behaves in any particular situation. Good mentors will also look out for experiences, or even create situations in which their mentees can become involved to learn new things, for example, providing a look behind the scenes or a glimpse at how other people live or do things.

3. **Be genuinely interested in your mentee as an individual**
    A mentoring relationship is a very personal one, which is often very important to the mentee, so, as a mentor, you need to get to know your mentee personally, about their hopes and dreams, so you can help them in a way that meets their personal best interest. For this reason, a parent is often not a good mentor for their child, as their parenting relationship and emotional connection will influence their guidance. That's not to say that a parent can never provide a mentoring moment for their child—they can—however, a parent can't be as objective as a person who's independent of the parenting role. In the same way, a manager is also not the best person to mentor someone on their team, as they'll often have a conflict of interest to contend with, between what's in the best interest of each individual and what's in the best interest of their team.

4. **Share your experiences and insights**
    In doing so, choose stories that you feel are appropriate and helpful, but do so in a neutral way, without any attachment to

Exhibit 5.2 *(Continued)*

how your mentee will use this learning. Be open to sharing your mistakes and failures too, as these are often where our biggest lessons are learned. It will also help your mentee be aware that challenges will arise, and the way you dealt with the situation might also help them gain insight about how to build resilience.

5. **Ask open questions**
Asking your mentee open questions will help you as a mentor to identify their real needs, values and passions. It's also a great way to get your mentee to think through situations themselves and draw out the consequences of the various choices or courses of action they can take. During these conversations, you can share your wisdom, without making decisions for your mentee. That's their job.

6. **Act as a sounding board**
Mentees benefit greatly from the opportunity of having a good mentor listen to them. Allow them to explore their thoughts and ideas openly with you. This will often help them unravel their thinking and gain insights about a situation as they share their concerns with you.

7. **Provide a fresh perspective**
One of the benefits of working with a mentor is that a good mentor will often provide their mentee with a fresh perspective on an issue. A good mentor will often have the clarity of distance from an issue or problem that's needed to provide objective feedback to their mentee. They can also hold up a 'mirror' to the mentee to, for example, let the mentee see what their behavior looks like to others.

8. **Provide helpful feedback**
Not all feedback is helpful. A good mentor knows this and will deliver feedback in a way that will help their mentee gain insight to further develop specific qualities or skills. For example, a good mentor will always ask for permission to give feedback before doing so. Giving unwelcome feedback can be detrimental to any mentoring relationship. Instead, explain what you'd like to talk about first and highlight the benefits of doing this.

(Continued on next page)

Exhibit 5.2 *(Continued)*

9. **Acknowledge achievements**

   Highlight for your mentee any achievements they might have forgotten, to help build their confidence. Remember to celebrate their successes on your mentoring journey too.

10. **Offer your advice, but only if your mentee asks for it**

    It can be very tempting for a mentor to just jump in and offer advice before a mentee has actually asked for it, especially when you've dealt with a similar situation yourself. Being a sounding board for your mentee, allowing them to discuss the situation with you, then helping them to think through the situation by asking them questions to draw out the consequences of various actions, is always more empowering for a mentee than advising them what to do. It helps them work through the issue and come to their own conclusions. By doing so, you ultimately help them to learn to think through issues themselves and trust their own judgment, both valuable life skills.

Source: Copyright © 2008. Used with permission from Blue Sky Coaching at www.blueskycoaching.com.au.

OVERCOMING BARRIERS TO MENTORING IN HEALTH SYSTEMS

Clearly, there is no shortage of insights into how to be an effective mentor. Why do we not see enough mentoring within health systems and hospital organizations?

The healthcare leaders interviewed for this text suggest common barriers to developing a culture that finds, develops, encourages, and rewards good mentors and good mentees. While the pressure rests more with the mentors to provide great mentoring than with the mentees to be proficient protégés, the mentees also have a responsibility to be open and responsive to the mentoring opportunity.

The five common obstacles include the following:

1. The organization's strategic and financial plan fails to acknowledge the essential power and importance of modern talent management (e.g., not only mentoring but also succession planning, continuity development of middle managers, and bold pay-for-performance programs) as an imperative for organizational growth and vitality. Explicit strategies and working capital to fund them must be formal components of the organization's short list of overall strategic imperatives.
2. The board of directors fails to communicate the expectation to the CEO that she is the chief champion for talent management systems and rewards in the organization's culture. The board must emphasize the importance it places on mentoring and leadership development among managers, physicians, nurses, and allied health professionals; request follow-up on progress; and celebrate gains made in the mentoring programs.
3. The CEO mandates the need for and value of mentoring but fails to serve as a mentor or does not intentionally seek to continuously develop and refine his own mentoring knowledge, skills, and attitudes. Even great CEOs need some encouragement to not only launch a serious mentoring initiative but also to stay with it over several years, and they must demonstrate a willingness and capacity to be a great mentor. The CEO must also encourage others on the senior executive team to seek and support mentoring throughout the organization.
4. Mentoring is viewed as the "flavor of the month" announced by senior managers and fails to be woven into the cultural fabric of the organization's performance management and incentive pay programs. Mentoring must be a durable and sustained part of the healthcare organization's DNA and continuously celebrated.

5. The mentoring imperative fails to assert the need for mentees to be fully engaged in and receptive to the organization's mentoring overtures. Mentees must be shown and continuously reminded that to be coached or mentored is not a sign that they are weak or poor performers. On the contrary, they are to feel flattered that the organization sees so much value and potential in them that it is willing to invest in their continuous growth and development. Leaders must instill the sincere belief in mentees that they are the future of the organization's growth and vitality and encourage them to be ready, willing, and able to participate fully and enthusiastically in the mentoring processes.

Executives may be reluctant to take on mentoring of the opposite sex, a situation in which the comfort level, socialization practices, and risk of appearing improper in this power differential dynamic can be a deterrent. Because the majority of CEOs are male, gender could serve as a barrier to protégée positions for women. As more and more of the graduates with advanced degrees in healthcare management entering the workforce are women who can benefit from mentoring experiences, strides must be made to overcome this additional barrier to mentoring in health systems.

As healthcare leaders map their strategies for a career of impact, they will find it helpful to develop strategies to overcome these obstacles to mentoring. Great leaders go even further, however; they embrace a positive, disciplined, multiyear commitment to mentor those around them. Only by developing others will we increase the prospects for our legacies to be powerful and long lasting.

THREE KEY ACTIONS TO HARDWIRE MENTORING INTO YOUR LEGACY ROAD MAP

Action 1: Make a commitment to reading eclectic material about mentoring in diverse industries.

Action 2: Ask a leader whom you respect to share ideas, experiences, and what he believes are essential ingredients to an effective and sustainable mentoring program.

Action 3: Work side-by-side with a mentee to define her career aspirations and interests, and create a brief road map for a multi-month mentoring experience to include
—competencies you both believe are important for success in the mentee's career path,
—a candid assessment of the competencies already possessed by the mentee that can be further cultivated and of those that are lacking, and
—specific strategies and learning opportunities to address these competency enhancement endeavors.

CHAPTER 6

Managing Diversity

LIVING WITH AND managing demographic diversity has become a central theme of the twenty-first century (Dunn 2010, 490). As a nation, the United States is ill prepared to deal with the challenges that new demographic trends present. Nowhere is this lack of preparation more critical than in healthcare, where failure to understand and appropriately care for demographically diverse patients exacerbates health disparities, increases the morbidity and mortality of large segments of our population, and significantly drives up the costs of healthcare (Schulte 2010, 1). Failure to understand and motivate a cross-cultural workforce will increasingly thwart the achievement of organizational goals and, in the process, derail a leader's career effectiveness. Creating, embracing, and sustaining a culture of diversity is essential to the success of healthcare legacy leaders.

Healthcare executives can no longer think of diversity only in terms of race and gender. We live in a multicultural society and do business in a global economy. Indeed, the Institute of Medicine reported in 2004 that "the United States is rapidly transforming into one of the most racially and ethnically diverse nations in the world" (IOM 2004, 23). Clearly, "the diversity challenges confronting leaders today are unlike those of just a decade ago" (Dunn 2010, 489).

> **"Diversity is good.** The challenge is how to bring its value to the organization.**"**
> —**Ed Dahlberg,** LFACHE

But how is diversity today different from the diversity of the past, how do we currently define diversity, and what challenges does the "new diversity" present for healthcare leaders?

CHANGE IS COMPLEX AND ACCELERATING

Several changes in our society over the last decade carry major implications for healthcare. If healthcare leaders do not take them into consideration, their organizations' success, and their leadership legacy, will be suboptimized.

Demographics

Armada and Hubbard (2010, 4), citing data from the US Census Bureau, note that "48 of the 100 largest cities in the United States have minority-majorities. Five states—California, Texas, Hawaii, New Mexico, and Florida—also have minority-majorities and five other states, including New York, are expected to become minority-majority soon." Furthermore, they write, from now until 2050, more than 90 percent of the population

> **Henry Ford Health System is a role model for diversity. Its Seven** Pillar Strategic Framework—people, service, quality and safety, growth, research and education, community, and finance—provides the foundation for the alignment of diversity goals, priorities, and metrics. We have integrated diversity into everything we do. We don't see challenges—we see opportunities.**
>
> **—Nancy M. Schlichting**

growth in the United States is projected to be people of color. As of 2011, one in six Americans is Hispanic (Venegas 2011).

Immigration Patterns

Reflecting shifts in immigration patterns, most immigrants to the United States now arrive from Eastern Europe, India, China, Southeast Asia, Africa, Mexico, and South America. Not only are the language, religion, and culture of these immigrants significantly different from the predominantly Western European immigrants of the past, but their views of illness and Western medicine are often dissimilar as well (Armada and Hubbard 2010, 12).

Another shift related to immigration is the nature of newcomers' goals upon arriving in the United States: Rather than aiming to assimilate into the "melting pot," as did many immigrants of the past, today people now immigrating often strive to preserve and celebrate the unique culture and way of life of these diverse countries of origin.

> **Diversity is in** our roots. I have diversity within my own family, so I don't see why it should be difficult to accept it within the workplace.**
>
> **—Ed Dahlberg,** LFACHE

> **Cultural issues** are unique to geographic areas. For example, the Hmong population in Minneapolis/ St. Paul is now active politically and has become a real force.**
>
> **—John G. King,** LFACHE

Laws and Regulations

Specific laws, regulations, and accrediting standards are in place to ensure diversity is honored and discrimination is eliminated. As in other areas of healthcare operations, legal and regulatory mandates for diversity bring increased complexity to healthcare management. Administrative attention must be given to ensure systematic, accurate patient data collection and that employee recruitment and hiring practices reflect the diversity of the patient population.

DRIVERS OF CHANGE

At one time, the human resources department was responsible for diversity initiatives, which were driven by equal employment opportunity laws and affirmative action practices and focused on race and gender to achieve a quota. Now, it is often clinicians who are driving the initiatives because of their concerns about misinterpreting diversity-related symptoms. For example, disease descriptions that are inaccurately understood can disrupt safety and quality of patient care (Armada and Hubbard 2010, 15).

Limited English Proficiency

Limited English proficiency (LEP) is now a prevalent-enough characteristic of the US population to have its own acronym. Twenty percent of US residents do not speak English at home; in some states, that figure is as high as 43 percent. These percentages do not include the 20 million individuals who are hearing impaired and use sign language or other means to communicate (Armada and Hubbard 2010, 9).

> **"The challenge in** working with diverse groups of employees is to understand how they interpret what it is that we are trying to do and how their backgrounds inform their understanding. Understanding their cultures and finding a balance [underlie] a terrific opportunity for the recruitment and training of needed employees.**"**
>
> **—Ed Dahlberg, LFACHE**

> **"As a general rule, it is the senior-level executive workforce** that is lacking in diversity. I think we have done pretty well at the intermediate level. Subsequent generations will benefit from this because the pipeline is reasonably well attended to.**"**
>
> **—David J. Fine, FACHE**

Sexual Orientation

Public conversations and political debate have brought the interests of openly lesbian, gay, bisexual, and transgender individuals to the forefront of demographic awareness. Indeed, the initialism LGBT is commonly recognized in management circles. This awareness is a significant driver of change in healthcare practices that will only increase in importance.

Global Economy

The US economy is wide open to global competition. This economic reality has in turn called attention to legal actions lodged against US-based multinational companies surrounding their failures to successfully integrate a diverse workforce. Healthcare is not immune to these failures. For example, the United Steelworkers union and the International Labor Rights Fund brought legal action against Coca-Cola alleging that Coca-Cola maintains relations with death squads to intimidate union leaders and repress trade union rights at its plants in Colombia. In another example, the National Labor Committee, *Businessweek*, and others have condemned Wal-Mart for sweatshop working conditions at its international factories. Wal-Mart's defense included that it conforms to local laws. But multicultural diversity brings differences in occupational safety and child labor laws, worker expectations, and business practices. US-based multinational organizations, including healthcare, must adhere to the laws and ethical standards of the United States.

Aging Workforce

The currently fragile economy and pending leadership shortages likely mean that many aging baby boomers will defer retirement and remain in C-suite positions, further increasing the generation gap between healthcare management and its workforce.

Increased Poverty

The socioeconomically disadvantaged experience a disproportionate burden of morbidity and mortality, and their numbers are increasing. Growing income inequalities will result in a rise in the numbers of uninsured and underinsured, who have less access to care.

Healthcare's Public Image

Healthcare organizations that fail to institute diversity initiatives may experience decreased patient satisfaction, lose market share, and risk future reimbursement. These predictions are especially valid if reimbursement becomes tied to patient satisfaction and outcomes (Armada and Hubbard 2010, 14).

> **"At Blue Cross/Blue** Shield Association, we worked with local MHA programs to establish diversity graduate fellowships. The payoff was our organization got the first pick of minority graduates for management.**"**
>
> —**Patrick G. Hays**, FACHE

International Medical Graduates

The number of international medical graduates (IMGs) working in the United States has been growing since 1981. Currently, more than 25 percent of US physicians are IMGs (Garman, Johnson, and Royer 2011), giving rise to potential cross-cultural conflicts among physicians, patients, and staff.

THE MANY FACES OF DIVERSITY

According to Armada and Hubbard (2010, 39), "diversity can be defined narrowly or broadly based on the unique attributes of a provider community and those stakeholders who are invested in the cultural, economic, and social life of an organization." The importance placed on diversity initiatives is directly related to the demographics of the population served.

As in the past, race and gender remain high on the diversity agenda, as they should. Women and people of color are most visibly underrepresented among minorities in healthcare management. In addition, today's multicultural society requires that leaders attend to several other groups on the diversity list. The implications for healthcare operations related to diversity among ethnic, cultural, generational, and religious groups as well as those with varied life experiences, economic status (including homelessness), sexual orientation, and disabilities are significant. Further complicating care delivery is the fact that an individual may be a member of more than one of these groups.

Finally, the healthcare environment is made more complex still by a multidisciplinary, multicultural healthcare workforce whose members bring their personal codes of conduct, values, and biases to the workplace.

> **Multicultural societies require multicultural organizations, and** multicultural organizations require multicultural leadership. It is the leadership where we have fallen short. The leadership must reflect the community that is served and must understand the employee population that is being managed.
> —**Thomas C. Dolan**, PhD, FACHE, CAE

> **Fellowships provide an organization with great recruitment** advantages. You are able to observe strengths and weaknesses, make better job offers, and reduce the chance of failure.
> —**David J. Fine**, FACHE

> **"A major challenge for healthcare organizations is that they are in** competition with corporations [that] have extensive in-house training opportunities for minority recruits. The ACHE Diversity Internship has been an attractive option for minority candidates.
>
> We need to hire more people who are different. This may mean expanding our definition of qualifications, being more flexible about markers of success, enhancing our educational opportunities.**"**
>
> **—Thomas C. Dolan, PhD, FACHE, CAE**

All of these diverse ingredients could be likened to a "demographic martini—shaken not stirred." But this reference to James Bond films may be lost on readers of later generations and from non-Western cultures. And therein lies the dilemma. Leaders can no longer assume that everyone shares their standards, values, sense of humor, and ways of thinking. We do not all see the world through the same lens. This reality has a significant impact not only on patient access, treatment, and outcomes but also on the outcomes of a leader's efforts. Healthcare executives must manage diversity in ways that ensure safe, high-quality care for patients and maintain harmony and collaboration among diverse staff. Workforce effectiveness and leadership success demand a sharp focus on understanding and leading diverse groups, organizations, and communities.

Heightened recognition of diversity and the issues it introduces into the healthcare management environment informs leadership actions and career effectiveness. The various components of diversity are presented in the following section. (This discussion is not intended to be a comprehensive look at the characteristics of diverse groups or the issues surrounding them, as much has been written elsewhere in that regard.)

> **"Don't hire just one minority. They need professional colleagues, too.** Also, be prepared to pay above market for good minority candidates. The demand is greater than the supply, so you must be highly competitive.**"**
>
> **—Patrick G. Hays, FACHE**

Race

Workforce

Racial minorities are still underrepresented in healthcare leadership positions. While it is accepted that leadership diversity should reflect that of the community being served, difficulties often arise in the recruitment and hiring of minorities. Healthcare leaders still grapple with the question of what factors should guide the hiring process: the qualifications and capabilities of the candidate, the organization's goal for diversity in leadership, or the personal preference of the hiring authority (Garman, Johnson, and Royer 2011, 123)?

> **"We have multi-disciplinary team–based diversity training for all staff at all levels. Through our education programs, we hard-wire sensitivity to differences into our service culture."**
>
> **—Nancy M. Schlichting**

In addition, healthcare organizations often find they must compete with other industries for bright, promising minority candidates, in part because the healthcare sector has underinvested in leadership training programs. If healthcare leaders expect to strengthen the breadth and depth of minority leadership, they must commit more time and resources to minority leadership development and mentoring programs.

Minority candidates must be hired for what they bring to the organization. Their employment should further the ambitions and goals of both the candidate and the organization. Well-advised healthcare leaders avoid "tokenism," foster inclusiveness, and expand mentoring and networking opportunities for minority managers. A leader's legacy road map must be designed to guide her through challenging and, in some cases, uncharted waters.

Patients

"Research has found that minority populations have a higher level of mistrust of healthcare providers," according to Hofmann (2010). And with good reason. Evidence confirms that racial and ethnic disparities exist in healthcare. Minority professionals are less visible to patients during the healthcare experience, and physicians of color have not always been recruited or welcomed by organizations (Hofmann 2010).

Failure to recognize cultural differences among racial minorities further hinders competent patient care. Cordova, Beaudin, and Iwanabe (2010, 23) found that the "healthcare industry has no standardized requirements for [data] collection, categorization, or use." Healthcare leaders need to strongly advocate for these standards to further enhance culturally competent care. Assumptions that all blacks are African American, for example, are simply incorrect. Many members of the black population are of Caribbean or South American descent with entirely different backgrounds and cultures than those of African Americans. Segments of the black population may also differ in their religion and language. Similar assumptions regarding those categorized as Asian Americans/Pacific Islanders (who comprise 43 ethnic groups with 100 different languages) and Hispanics must be avoided (Cordova, Beaudin, and Iwanabe 2010, 36). The term *Hispanic* was introduced by the US Census Bureau in the 1980s as a way to categorize people connected to the Spanish language; it conveys no meaning regarding race or national origin. Hispanics may be black or white and may originate from more than 20 countries.

> **"Our multicultural society presents recruitment challenges, but** they are challenges that can be met. Success depends on the kinds of staff that you are looking for. We do a decent job of recruiting professional and technical staff but not so well at the executive and management levels. We don't know the true sources of supply for these candidates. The traditional sources of supply, like university programs, don't have the diversity we need. Because of other pressing challenges, we won't or can't spend the resources or the effort finding new sources of supply.
>
> Promoting from within doesn't improve our odds of getting diversity. We need to broaden our scope beyond healthcare—look at other industries and where they find diverse candidates. Some corporations have had programs in place for 15–20 years, and diversity recruitment is part of their MBO [management by objectives] program.**"**
>
> **—Donald C. Wegmiller, FACHE**

Culture and Ethnicity

Legacy leaders appreciate that we live and work in a multicultural world. Dunn (2010, 490) states, "Culture is the sum total of one's way of living [and] includes values, beliefs, standards, language, thinking patterns, behavioral norms, communication styles, and other background and experience factors." All of these influences guide an individual's decisions and actions. Failure to recognize this aspect of human nature by treating all people the same, known as "cultural blindness" (Dunn, 2010, 490), is sure to damage a leader's legacy.

Data Collection

Data collection to measure diversity by both the US Census Bureau and healthcare organizations is unreliable. Cultural and ethnic categories are vague and general, variances in self-identification and reluctance of data collectors to verify their own assumptions increase inaccuracies, and data collection does not take country of origin into account. An Institute of Medicine (2000, 294) report assessing health communication strategies for diverse populations suggests that data collection for diversity should be reformulated as a sociocultural process. This approach would identify individuals specifically by culture, customs, and language rather than by skin color or continent of origin. Such a method makes sense, considering one of the more significant barriers to culturally competent care is language.

Patients

Armada and Hubbard (2010, 3) write, "Cross-cultural healthcare involves three key issues: racial and ethnic disparities in quality of care provided in minority patients; cross-cultural value differences between immigrant patients and Western medical providers; and providing language assistance to limited and disabled persons." They contend that the goal of cultural competency training is to "create a healthcare system and workforce that are capable of delivering the highest quality of care to every patient regardless of race, ethnicity, culture, or language proficiency" (Armada and Hubbard 2010, 13). According to Cordova, Beaudin, and Iwanabe (2010, 20), the cultural competency of an organization can be measured by "its capacity to integrate principles and values of cultural competence into its policy, structure, attitudes, behaviors, and practices." How must healthcare leaders master these challenges as they earn, inspire, engage, and partner with followers?

LEP and disabled patients are guaranteed the right to language assistance access by law. Healthcare facilities that participate in Medicare and Medicaid are legally bound to provide language assistance. For guidance in ensuring compliance, hospitals and health systems may turn to The Joint Commission and the National Quality Forum, which offer cultural competency standards for patients' access to language accommodation.

In addition to adhering to laws and regulations, providing language assistance makes good business sense. Hispanics, the largest minority in the United States, frequently choose hospitals on the basis of the level of language assistance provided. Providing language assistance reduces poor communication, medical errors, and healthcare costs. For example, costs escalate because physicians tend to order more diagnostic tests and hospital admissions when they cannot communicate adequately with the patient or family (Armada and Hubbard 2010, 9, 10).

Progressive healthcare organizations provide language accommodations. For example, Children's Hospital Los Angeles offers interpreters in 33 languages around the clock, pictorial communication materials for the illiterate, and a website in the languages of its community. Children's Hospital Central California added a telephone line for patients to access discharge instructions in three languages (Cordova, Beaudin, and Iwanabe 2010, 26–28).

Finally, ensuring that health communications with diverse patients and family members are clear and well understood is an ethical mandate. The guiding principles in the ethical treatment of patients include respecting an individual's autonomy, providing benefit, avoiding harm, and treating groups and individuals justly and equitably. These tenets cannot be fulfilled unless patients, families, and caregivers can communicate clearly (Institute of Medicine 2000, 305).

Workforce

The multicultural workforce brings its own set of considerations to the attention of healthcare leaders. As with patients, employees must be treated justly and equitably. And as with patients, communications must be clear and well understood if the work is to get done and the desired goals achieved.

Dunn (2010, 491) cites four challenges in managing multicultural teams of employees: differences in communication style, differences in attitudes toward hierarchy and authority, difficulty understanding accents and low-fluency speech, and conflicting norms for decision making. For example, people from non-Western cultures typically use indirect communication, prefer to communicate with those of the same culture, and discuss decisions at length, while individuals from Western cultural backgrounds tend to communicate directly, make decisions quickly, and not dwell on those decisions once they are made. These style differences can impede staff collaboration and harmony. Healthcare leaders must be able to mobilize and influence multicultural teams who may be very different from themselves to live the organization's mission and achieve its goals.

Gender

Despite the fact that large numbers of women complete university graduate programs in health services administration and many women serve in middle management healthcare positions, women continue to be underrepresented in senior leadership and governance positions.

> **❝I advise younger women to only work in organizations that want** you to be there, that value your leadership, and where you can truly make a contribution.❞
>
> —Nancy M. Schlichting

> **❝Throughout my career, I have been purposefully disproportionate** in the number of fellowships for minorities and women that we offer. This is at least partially due to the need to counterbalance the historically fraternal aspects of the healthcare C-suite.❞
>
> —David J. Fine, FACHE

The "glass ceiling," that invisible but real barrier to women rising to the highest ranks of management, persists as an obstacle to optimal organizational performance and talent development. Observers offer a variety of reasons for its persistence. Some claim that the image of leaders as male is deeply embedded in the American psyche. The fact that women have held high positions in other countries, such as Britain's Margaret Thatcher, India's Indira Ghandi, and Germany's Angela Merkel, suggests that this image issue is unique to the United States. Others say subtle and frustrating gender discrimination is at play. Still others contend the glass ceiling is a function of organizational structure, a systemic flaw that prevents women from rising to the top. Regardless of the reason, many healthcare organizations continue to forgo opportunities to benefit from a valuable female talent pool. Those led by enlightened leaders, on the other hand, seek out, mentor, and develop women leaders because they bring an important perspective and set of skills to the executive team. Modern legacy leaders make certain that their organizations provide equal compensation for women, afford equal access to information for effective decision making, and tolerate no sexual discrimination or harassment. They seek to eliminate structural barriers to the advancement of women managers, and they place women on teams and in positions where they may gain knowledge and experience needed to grow in their careers. Above all, legacy leaders trust and expect women executives to perform as successfully as their male counterparts do.

The Generation Divide

Patricia Crown, PhD, distinguished professor in the Department of Anthropology at the University of New Mexico, shared this experience regarding generation differences: In the past she would refer to the concentric circles on a record album to describe ancient pottery until her students asked, "What's a record album?"

How can leaders be effective if they cannot connect with their teams, staff, and communities, all of which are composed of members of several generations? More to the point, how can leaders achieve a career of impact if they suboptimize their engagement with followers by being inattentive to generational trends, knowledge, and ways of thinking?

Workforce

What once was the "generation gap" has become the "generation divide," a gulf that has been widened by new communication styles and technologies. The generations entering the workforce today prefer to text rather than talk, and they obtain information from

> "Ethnicity remains the biggest issue in diversity. People of color are a visual difference. Gender is still a major issue as well. Younger women really don't know what older women experienced."
>
> —Thomas C. Dolan, PhD, FACHE, CAE

> "Whether we like it or not, my observation is people coming up the ranks in health administration march to a different drummer. Many in earlier generations thought of health administration as a calling—they felt called to serve people—hence the term *servant leadership*. I don't see that so much anymore."
>
> —Patrick G. Hays, FACHE

> **"I admire the younger generation. They don't see gender, race, or** sexual orientation. They are more open-minded and more community oriented. They look at the world differently. We need to prepare more of this generation for leadership positions."
>
> —Nancy M. Schlichting

an Internet search engine instead of the library. Communication within this generation is most often informal, direct, and grammatically incorrect. Its members interact less often through human contact and more often via avatars (virtual persons); they operate less with a workbook and more with Facebook. These employees are more concerned with social justice, the environment, and family life than are their parents.

Leaders need to consider new ways to motivate and effectively communicate with this younger generation of employees. Its ranks are accustomed to acting on their own inclinations, so new-employee orientation programs must include, and explain the rationale for, rules of employment, professional conduct, business communication, dress, punctuality, and teamwork. Incentive and reward programs need to be oriented to what younger employees consider important benefits and perquisites—which will not include seniority in the organization.

According to a study by the University of New Mexico's Anderson School of Management, 70 percent of employers surveyed face some intergenerational conflict in the workplace. Their response is not surprising when you consider that, for the first time in history, four generations of employees may be working together in their organizations (Quigley 2011). Especially in healthcare, which is characterized by a great breadth and depth of education and skills throughout the workforce, leaders are challenged to bring generations together to share goals and knowledge and to "play well with others." Legacy leaders intentionally assign intergenerational teams to work on projects or initiatives and encourage generations to appreciate the experiences and skills they can share with each other. Mentoring across diverse groups of mentees, while adding complexity to a leader's effectiveness, is also recommended to bridge the workforce generation divide.

Patients

Emerging generational differences in the patient population require healthcare leaders and their teams to adopt new ways of communicating with patients and new services to meet those patients' needs. Leaders must implement marketing strategies using social networking and peer pressure to attract young adult patients and influence their decision making. Members of this age group have a community and group mind-set and visit community centers, participate in "Mommy" groups, and arrange play dates for their kids. The younger generations of patients are less likely to develop relationships with their physicians and more likely to rely on the Internet for their health information, much of which is unregulated. Healthcare leaders who develop Internet-accessible, current, reliable, and culturally appropriate health information for their communities will have a market edge.

As evidence of this trend, the *American Medical News* reported in late 2010 that 871 hospitals maintained more than 2,250 total social media sites, such as on Facebook and Twitter, to communicate with patients and physicians. Furthermore, hospitals are hiring staff specialists to manage social media and oversee their social media presence (Cook 2010).

The expanding older generations of patients present their own challenges, especially the growing numbers of people age 85 or above. This group presents with the most complex health problems and social support needs. Healthcare leaders need to develop innovative programs and services to support healthy aging at home and reduce costly hospitalizations (Garman, Johnson, and Royer 2011, 34).

Whether in terms of patients or employees, regardless of the differences between generations, healthcare leaders should remember that all people want to be treated with dignity and respect and typically will respond in kind.

Multicultural Professionals

Under the best circumstances, healthcare leaders face challenges in bringing medical staff on board; physicians typically focus on individual patients and are reluctant to commit time to an organization and to expending effort that may not bring immediate results. To promote diversity among the professional ranks, we recommend encouraging physicians in management positions to champion the organization's diversity initiatives with their colleagues. For this approach to succeed, however, executives must make sure physician managers witness and communicate to their colleagues the value—to them and their patients—of supporting diversity and actively participating in cultural competency education. Physicians, nurses, and other professionals must see the clinical benefit and recognize that diversity education is a good use of their time and not just "a nice thing to do."

Once they have successfully recruited diverse professionals, healthcare leaders must be ready to overcome the next layer of challenges posed by a multicultural medical staff. With IMGs constituting more than 25 percent of physicians practicing in the United States (Garman, Johnson, and Royer 2011, 43), the cultural values and attitudes they bring to the healthcare environment sometimes interfere with their ability to relate appropriately to patients or to

> "Healthcare leaders will be challenged to make certain that their minority patients, employees, and medical staff have equal experiences with their nonminority counterparts."
>
> —John G. King, LFACHE

> "Different cultures bring different values to the workplace. Physicians coming from cultures with class distinctions may have their behaviors in dealing with servants cross over into their hospital-based practice. This can present problems when attempting collaboration with nurses. 'Unlearning' of behaviors is sometimes in order, especially in physician executive programs when it becomes apparent that different styles will achieve better results."
>
> —David J. Fine, FACHE

> **When you have a diverse medical staff, they are more sensitive** to differences, so there is less conflict, not more. When you have diversity as an organizational strategy and leadership is aligned to it, you mitigate the risk of cross-cultural conflict.
>
> —Nancy M. Schlichting

collaborate with nurses and other caregivers. This dissonance may be especially prevalent for those whose countries of origin have class distinctions or different attitudes about the role of women. Hofmann (2011) says that "compounding the growing challenge of effectively caring for our multicultural society is the largely ignored influence of patients who trigger moral judgments by physicians, nurses and other clinicians." Such judgments can influence patient communication, treatment, and outcomes, so physicians need to understand their biases and how they may affect patient care. Note, however, that, some African-American healthcare professionals may express resentment of the attention and accommodations given to newer immigrant patients because this same concern was not readily offered black patients in the past (Armada and Hubbard 2010, 15). Thus, it behooves healthcare executives to attend to all the implications of their organization's diversity initiatives.

Physicians, for their part, must recognize the serious clinical issues associated with this new diversity. They need to understand not only the cultural differences surrounding death and dying, blood, transplants, mental health, and other potentially sensitive areas but also the diseases commonly seen in certain races and ethnic groups and those that are endemic to certain parts of the world. In addition, they must be able to interact effectively across cultures and work with interpreters (Armada and Hubbard 2010, 13–14).

Relationships between patients and caregivers significantly influence health outcomes, so it follows that diversity in the health professions that reflects the community improves patient satisfaction and compliance. However, the lack of availability of racially and ethnically diverse professionals to meet this need is problematic.

Current trends indicate that minority clinical professionals still face high barriers to entry into such segments as medicine, dentistry, and pharmacy (Cordova, Beaudin, and Iwanabe 2010, 22). Legacy leaders champion efforts to eliminate these barriers. (Refer to the excerpts from our interviews with the quoted leaders placed throughout this chapter for more insight into launching such efforts.)

The medical profession in the United States recognizes the need for its physicians to adapt to a multicultural society. In 2004, the Association of American Medical Colleges began requiring medical schools to teach cross-cultural medicine. As of 2006, three states—California, New Jersey, and Washington—require training in cross-cultural medicine to be granted licensure (Armada and Hubbard 2010, 12).

Sexual Orientation

As mentioned earlier, LGBT individuals have seen a shift in awareness of their concerns and needs. Although the topic of sexual orientation may elicit strong responses from some individuals and groups in the healthcare workplace and tensions may arise between heterosexual and gay employees, LGBT patients and staff warrant the same considerations as those afforded all other groups. Healthcare leaders will need to address sensitive issues related to sexual orientation, about which conflicting viewpoints may be expressed. They must be able to set aside any personal biases, hone their conflict management skills, and sharpen those communication skills that ferret out and address underlying causes of conflict.

> **The biggest challenge in** diversity management is for executives to understand and appreciate the differences and the different points of view that diversity brings to the organization.
>
> **—Thomas C. Dolan,**
> **PhD, FACHE, CAE**

Religious Faith and Beliefs

Many healthcare organizations were founded by faith-based organizations and have historically served a predominantly Christian population. As the United States has transitioned to a multicultural society, other faiths and beliefs have entered the healthcare landscape. Interdenominational chapels adorned with the crucifix may be an architectural artifact. Just as prayer in schools has become a topic for debate, conversations about how and what spiritual comfort is provided for patients and families will undoubtedly occur. And as with sexual orientation, strong emotions will accompany these discussions. Among the questions that intentionally aware leaders address are, Will caregivers bring their prejudices and biases to the bedside? Will the growing Muslim population be treated with the same respect and dignity as are members of the Christian population? How will the different beliefs of the Mormon,

> **"Many of our hospitals founded by religious orders must serve** non-Christians as well as Christians. There will be a question of how good they are at reaching the growing Muslim population.
>
> Managing diversity must start with the board and top management, whose composition must represent their minority communities. Efforts must be intentional, promoted with sensitivity, and motivated to seek richness of experience.**"**
>
> —**John G. King,** LFACHE

> **"As the crisis in the Middle East continues and the US Muslim** population increases, we may have to rethink the term *nondenominational* as applied to hospital chapels and give more thought to reasonable accommodations. There are no easy answers.**"**
>
> —**Thomas C. Dolan,** PhD, FACHE, CAE

Jew, Buddhist, Christian Scientist, and Confucian be honored? What about the agnostic? The atheist? As with other cultural differences, healthcare leaders must acquire sufficient knowledge and understanding of religions and beliefs to promote culturally competent care and to engender a productive and patient-centered workplace.

OPPORTUNITIES FOR HEALTHCARE LEADERS IN THE DIVERSITY ARENA

As a microcosm of the increasingly multicultural society, the US healthcare system must pay attention and respond to the needs of the new diversity of key stakeholders.

Governance and Leadership

Legacy leaders see opportunity in diversity. They harness their power to make diversity work to the advantage of the organization and the patients served. But they also must *value* diversity in the workplace—not just tolerate it, but truly appreciate it for the innovation it brings to the organization (Kouzes and Posner 1993, 95).

Grant (2010, 41) notes that "leadership representation, organizational culture, and organizational support of diversity are the most powerful change agents and should be the primary focus of diversity initiatives." In other words, diversity in the organization is leadership driven. Leadership must visibly support diversity initiatives and model them for the entire organization if the programs are to be taken seriously. The importance of diversity must be routinely included in leadership conversations. Legacy leaders champion advancement of diverse healthcare providers and managers and thereby promote organizational vitality.

As indicated earlier, the composition of leadership and the governing board should represent the community's demographic diversity. To achieve this representation, leaders must be proactive and persistent in recruiting minority members to serve in these roles. Governing boards must be held responsible to see that their membership appropriately reflects and is responsive to the community and should be encouraged to advance diversity initiatives within the organization. Cordova, Beaudin, and Iwanabe (2010,

❝I see four principal management challenges for healthcare leaders.

The first is to take at least partial responsibility for addressing the well-documented disparities in the health status as well as the healthcare outcomes of specific ethnic and minority populations.

The second is to assure the organization's diversity mirrors the community's to the greatest extent possible. In practical terms, this means the complexion of the governing body, senior management, medical staff, supervisory staff, and volunteers ideally should be comparable to that of the communities served by the organization.

The third is to help the above groups achieve not only cultural sensitivity but also cultural competency.

The fourth is to establish realistic but ambitious objectives and timelines to measure progress in each of the first three areas.❞

—Paul B. Hofmann, DrPH, FACHE

21) write, "The importance of the governing body's role in ensuring quality of care is increasing as public reporting of quality data becomes more prevalent and providing culturally equitable care is a safety issue."

Workforce

Workforce diversity presents multiple challenges for healthcare leaders. Executives must recognize the game-changing nature of expanded diversity and mobilize people of many different cultures, languages, and values to enhance organizational performance by sharing knowledge and experiences and by valuing each other's perspectives. Leaders will direct these efforts toward finding common ground in the mission of the organization and in the achievement of its goals.

Deciding how to communicate with, motivate, mentor, evaluate, and reward employees of different cultures requires forethought. Images, humor, and words carry different meanings to different cultures. Managers must be educated in cultural awareness and sensitivity to effectively manage their employees, and professional staff and caregivers must be trained to provide culturally competent care.

One advantage that diversity brings to an organization is the thoughtful dissent that can arise from multiple perspectives. It also enhances creativity, idea generation, productivity, and appreciation

> **"In seeking to better understand diversity, I have found personal** immersion to be most helpful for me: going to meetings where I'm the only minority; reaching out to groups who are not like me and spending time with them. Healthcare executives who are pressed for time might consider spending time in their departments with diverse populations of employees, like the laundry, or attending a black church or working with community groups of minority populations.**"**
>
> **—Thomas C. Dolan, PhD, FACHE, CAE**

for the perceptions of others. Hesselbein and Shrader (2008, 348) recommend assigning accountability for building a richly diverse team to every person who directs the work of others.

The new diversity of the workforce brings a variety of value systems to the workplace. Legacy leaders ensure clarity about rules of professionalism, employment, and standards of ethical conduct within their organizations.

Furthermore, successful healthcare leaders recognize and celebrate the importance of the demographic composition of the workforce. Employees, including visible caregivers, should reflect and respect the population being served because that reflection will aid recruitment and retention: The organization becomes attractive to potential candidates, not to mention consumers of healthcare, when its workforce looks, sounds, and acts like them.

At a recent BridgeWorks conference, participants were advised to prepare for the coming worker shortage. Within seven years, the presenters projected, 30 million currently employed workers will be over the age of 55. To mitigate a potential leadership drain, healthcare organizations need to develop new leaders now from a multicultural generation, which comes with all the different values and ambitions discussed in this chapter (Lancaster and Stillman 2011). Successful legacy leaders have the vision to plan accordingly and recognize that, to be an employer of choice, their organizations must find a talented employee pool now and keep it in the future.

Patient Population

As implied through this chapter, healthcare leaders today must ensure that the multicultural patient population they serve receives culturally competent and safe care. According to Cordova, Beaudin, and Iwanabe (2010, 20), the cultural competency of an organization can be measured by "its capacity to integrate principles and values of cultural competence into its policy, structures, attitudes, behaviors, and practices." To accomplish this integration, effective legacy leaders adopt a systems approach to diversity and develop diversity initiatives as part of the strategic direction, including all facets of strategic planning and decision-making processes.

Healthcare executives must also make sure that the commitment to culturally competent care permeates the entire organization and the entire workforce (Cordova, Beaudin, and Iwanabe 2010, 23). Such widespread commitment requires ongoing staff education at all levels of the organization that is based on patient data and immigration patterns of the service area. Sharing knowledge derived from case studies and grand rounds works well in educating clinicians and is a key component to mentoring and developing managers.

THE BUSINESS CASE FOR DIVERSITY

Legacy leaders know their communities—not just their demographic patterns but also the people, with all their unique cultural needs and expectations, who populate those communities. To better understand the community, healthcare leaders need to build creative partnerships with civic organizations, schools, religious organizations, and cultural groups that represent it. Legacy leaders are not just observers; they are participants in efforts that affect the health and well-being of those they serve. Examples of such efforts include enlightened public policy, advocacy, health promotion activities, and dissemination of healthcare career information.

The American College of Healthcare Executives, American Hospital Association, Association of American Medical Colleges, Catholic Health Association of the United States, and National Association of Public Hospitals and Health Systems have joined to pursue the goal of eliminating health disparities and improving the quality of care for every patient. These organizations ask healthcare executives to fully embrace three key practices: increase the collection and use of race, ethnicity, and language preference data; increase cultural competency training; and increase diversity in governance and management.

In 2011, the Health Research & Educational Trust (HRET) and the Institute for Diversity in Health Management (IFD) published "Building a Culturally Competent Organization: The Quest for Equity in Health Care." The publication presents the indisputable case for action on the diversity front. Of course, culturally competent healthcare can be advocated on the grounds that it is politically correct, socially correct, and ethically correct, but as minorities

"Diversity can be defined in so many ways. We need to use our resources carefully and choose programs where we can show some success quickly and dramatically. The most visible minorities remain those of color.**"**

—**Patrick G. Hays, FACHE**

"We focus on diversity in everything we do—this includes supplier diversity. It is who we are as an organization and who we are as a community.**"**

—**Nancy M. Schlichting**

become an increasingly large proportion of the US population, cultural competency in healthcare becomes a business requirement and a clinical necessity as well. In fact, it can be said that the health and productivity of the nation depend on the ability of our healthcare organizations to deliver culturally competent care. HRET and IFD (2011, 2–3) identify seven tasks, with accompanying self-assessment questions, for healthcare leaders to move their organizations in the direction of representational diversity:

1. Collect race, ethnicity, and language preference
2. Identify and report disparities
3. Provide culturally and linguistically competent care
4. Develop culturally competent disease management programs
5. Increase diversity and minority workforce pipelines
6. Involve the community
7. Make cultural competency an institutional priority

The HRET/IFD report also reminds us that laws and regulations are in place that support culturally competent care. These include Title VI of the Civil Rights Act of 1964; the US Department of Health and Human Services National Standards on Culturally and Linguistically Appropriate Services; relevant Joint Commission accreditation standards; Executive Order 13166, "Improving Access to Services for Persons with Limited Language Proficiency"; and the 2010 Patient Protection and Affordable Care Act. Healthcare leaders must be knowledgeable about these laws and regulations and ensure that their organizations are in compliance (HRET and IFD 2011, 6).

Some states have also undertaken initiatives to move their healthcare organizations closer to diversity standards. The New Mexico Department of Health, in partnership with the Agency for Healthcare Research and Quality, is improving the New Mexico Hospital Inpatient Discharge Data to increase the quality, completeness, and reliability of the state's race and ethnicity data. All nonfederal hospitals across the state are implementing a standardized collection method based on the 1997 Office of Management and Budget Standards for the Classification of Federal Data on Race and Ethnicity and launching a program of extensive data collection for Native American tribal affiliates. This effort acknowledges the need for healthcare leaders to know their state and local populations and implement programs according to their makeup. New Mexico serves as a good example of how diversity affects healthcare delivery: Its Native American population is large and brings tribal differences to the healthcare arena that must be accommodated to ensure safe and effective care for the community.

> **"Exceptional senior leadership and the design and implementation** of clear incentives are indispensable in motivating appropriate organizational behavior. Effective management should produce more innovative programs to improve intervention efforts, educational initiatives, recruitment activities, and training courses. Successful strategies that deal with this new diversity will depend on acquiring and maintaining reliable data and establishing new community partnerships. However, sustainable progress will be unlikely unless designated executives are held accountable for specific issues and significant accomplishments are properly celebrated.**"**
>
> **—Paul B. Hofmann, DrPH, FACHE**

THREE KEY ACTIONS TO HARDWIRE DIVERSITY INTO YOUR LEGACY ROAD MAP

Action 1: Be intentional about ensuring that leaders and trustees reflect the diversity of the community they serve. Commit to strategies for diversity recruitment and retention, and make certain that these efforts translate throughout the organization.

Action 2: Commit to learning about and understanding your multicultural patient population through personal immersion and community partnerships.

Action 3: Commit your organization to delivering culturally competent, safe patient care. Review and complete the HRET/IFD (2011) self-assessment questions, and use the feedback to implement programs that address organizational needs currently going unfulfilled. Research successful staff education and LEP programs in support of this legacy road map action step.

CHAPTER 7

Leading Innovation

INNOVATION HAS BECOME a core driver of growth, performance, and value (Barsh, Capozzi, and Davidson 2008). As the importance of innovation grows, conventional wisdom needs to be replaced with "innovational wisdom," that is, applied knowledge that is continuously reviewed, refined, and renewed to drive the behavior of the leadership team and its organizational units.

Leaders who make a positive difference in the operations and culture of high-performing organizations exhibit innovation leadership in part by rarely procrastinating and frequently challenging the status quo. These traits demonstrate innovational wisdom and allow organizations to be nimble competitors by attracting patient, payer, and donor support.

This chapter reveals innovation strategies to improve services and performance. It also provides guidance on how to frame questions and address challenges through a fresh perspective, especially for leaders from clinical backgrounds, such as physicians, nurses, and allied health professionals.

INNOVATION LEADERSHIP

Just as fulfilling stakeholders' demands for superior healthcare and value requires continuous analysis of organizational strengths, weaknesses, opportunities, and threats, plotting one's career of impact requires the periodic review and refinement of one's legacy road map. This dual analysis generates crucial innovations in both the organization and the leader's career. But how does one translate this knowledge to innovation leadership? Legacy leaders master and champion innovation as a concept and encourage innovation all the time, everywhere.

Legacy Leaders Master and Champion Innovation

Leading innovation requires visionary purpose and the establishment of stretch, or audacious, goals. Colleagues look to healthcare leaders to champion fresh ways of looking at old, persistent challenges, and legacy leaders see this demonstration of followership as an opportunity to practice innovation.

Legacy Leaders Encourage Innovation All the Time, Everywhere

Legacy leaders can find many practical ways to understand and apply innovation in their journey to a career of impact. For example, Rosabeth Moss Kanter (1997, 7) suggests we deploy "idea scouts" to look for ideas beyond the organization and industry.

Several of the healthcare leaders interviewed for this book's exploration of legacy road maps assert that to be innovative occasionally is a reasonably attainable objective, but to continuously be innovative is not easy. It requires a disciplined set of leadership attributes, including the following:

- An intense curiosity about alternate solutions
- An avid interest in reading eclectic literature on design thinking and problem solving in other industries
- A willingness to encourage, enable, and empower staff to take sensible risks to redefine the problem and rethink the solutions

Legacy leaders apply these traits to bringing an innovation culture to their organizations.

SOCIAL INNOVATION

Collins (1997) encourages leaders to shift their attention from innovative products and technology to "social innovation." How can legacy leaders become what Collins calls "social inventors"? Leaders practice social innovation by consistently fostering a culture in which staff are hungry for fresh thinking, are eager to map new approaches to old challenges, and engage in collaborative teamwork whereby team members are not afraid to propose any idea—even an idea that initially may seem outrageous.

Similar to social inventors, leaders who follow a structured legacy road map are more likely than others to create organizational cultures that encourage continuous improvement, sensible risk taking, and innovation. The healthcare leaders interviewed for this book agree, as reflected in their excerpted quotes throughout the text.

UNLEASHING INNOVATION

Legacy leaders unleash innovation throughout the organization by creating a high-performance culture. How do you create such a culture? By adhering to the following rules (Robbins 2007, 3):

1. Be outcome oriented.
2. Be feedback rich.
3. Create a balanced approach to management that gives people the motivation to move forward and a vision (and a pathway) to achieve success.
4. Know yourself.
5. Coach others.
6. Push for those ideas that will change the way you operate.

To further strengthen the innovation culture at your organization, convene several staff members once per quarter for a "3i Lab" (ideas, insights, initiatives) session. The session should cover the following three questions:

1. What are the big challenges we see as holding back our pursuit of excellence?
2. What are the two to three bold new ideas that could help us remove or work around these challenges?
3. What initiatives should we take to ensure these ideas happen, take root, and flourish?

Morris contends that leaders will be more likely to sustain such a culture if they implement all of the following characteristics for top-down innovation (Morris 2011):

1. *Attitude.* A legacy leader's demeanor inspires passion for innovation and the teamwork to pursue it.
2. *Expectations.* Legacy leaders not only share their expectation for innovation frequently and across all segments of the organization but also model those expectations in their daily behavior.
3. *Policy.* Most organizational policy contexts—from hiring to incentive pay to board agendas to medical staff meetings to purchasing to patient safety to revenue cycle management to annual performance reviews—must encourage and enable the above-mentioned expectations.
4. *Strategy.* In essence, a legacy leader's strategy is innovation and his innovations are strategic. Your staff know what you value by how you allocate your time. They will follow your lead if you invest your time and energy on optimizing strategies for innovation.
5. *Enablers.* Healthcare leaders should trust their staff to take risks and implement an innovation process by which they can creatively take those risks.

Furthermore, staff must know that leaders trust them to take such risks and understand the purpose of the process that is in place to foster innovation.

Innovation without methodology is luck. If intentionally given the chance, the creative people in your healthcare organization will innovate. But if an organization relies on random efforts, it risks its future success on chance. The Mayo Clinic Center for Innovation (www.mayo.edu/center-for-innovation/) suggests developing and applying "design thinking" methodologies to make the shift from luck to consistency, predictability, and sustainability. For healthcare delivery, design thinking means redesigning the patient experience by vigorously challenging traditional ways of building care delivery venues, providing disease management, and offering top value (Center for Innovation 2012).

6. *Removing obstacles*. Legacy leaders work diligently to remove the key obstacles—behavioral, organizational, and methodological—to innovation.

Behavioral obstacles can range from team members' unwillingness to entertain ideas from another organization to fears that change will constrain a middle manager's prerogatives to anxiety about an unknown future, all of which build resistance to change. Legacy leaders break through such behavior constraints by articulating a desirable future state (a vision) and/or creating the burning platform.

Organizational obstacles can range from a lack of information or expertise to fuel the pursuit of new methods and mind-sets to a lack of working capital to support the innovations.

Legacy leaders engage with their colleagues and staff to build bridges from the current organizational structures and culture to a more accommodating environment that yields early wins and pride with new results.

Methodological obstacles often manifest themselves in a lack of prior experience with the innovative processes or designs, and a lack of experience in the science of what the

Center for Innovation (2012) refers to as "design thinking." Legacy leaders build into their road map planning, consideration of design thinking, and creation of cultures of constant inquiry that foster an impatience with the status quo and a hunger for continuous improvement.

INNOVATION LABS EXPRESS CULTURE

Kaiser Permanente and Mayo Clinic consider innovation to be an imperative for organizational vitality and longevity. These high-performing health systems have invested millions of dollars in developing cultures of continuous improvement. This investment supports interdisciplinary, hands-on practice labs through which the organizations apply design thinking to champion and facilitate innovation.

Kaiser and Mayo also foster intangible components of innovation, an interesting and perhaps unexpected mix of curiosity, evidence-based design, and willingness to celebrate risk and failure in service to patient-centered performance enhancements.

How a leader manages failure is key to an innovation culture. Sloane (2012) proposes three key steps that organizations must take—and effectively communicate to their employees—to create an atmosphere in which failure is not only respected but encouraged:

1. Distinguish between the two kinds of failure:
   • Honorable failure
   • Incompetent failure
2. Allow people the freedom to fail.
3. Celebrate honorable failures as well as sustainable successes.

For example, in patient safety, an honorable failure made in pursuit of innovation would be a nursing unit's recognition that the design for a new nurses station failed to adequately accommodate space for confidential review with physicians of a patient's behavior changes from a new medication regimen. A sustainable success would be reduced medication errors as a result of a new initiative to scan patient ID bracelet bar codes to verify individual medication orders.

We provide clinical examples above, but healthcare leadership also is ripe for this kind of innovation. To fulfill a career of impact, leaders need to embed innovation into their legacy road maps.

Govindarajan and Peters (2011), in writing about the success General Electric (GE) has experienced through its Leadership, Innovation and Growth program, share the following factors crucial to innovation leadership, which healthcare leaders can hardwire into their legacy road maps:

1. Keep intact teams together for development.
2. Secure leadership support.
3. Leverage actionable frameworks.
4. Create a common language.
5. Conduct extensive follow-up.
6. As successes emerge, share best practices to maintain the momentum of what has been learned and to drive further adoption across the hospital or health system.

These six actions reinforce the team's pride of accomplishment and demonstrate that the organization is professional and persistent in its pursuit of innovation throughout the organization.

To encourage the entire leadership team to adopt these guidelines, legacy leaders, operating with disciplined processes for unleashing innovation opportunities, place individuals in a variety of roles, as depicted in McKinsey & Company's innovation network (Exhibit 7.1) (Barsh, Capozzi, and Davidson 2008). Through this model, it is clear that an individual innovator cannot generate enough momentum to effect change; the organization needs a network of innovators functioning within a clearly defined infrastructure and including four types of leaders/staff:

1. *Idea generators*, who are willing to take risks on high-profile experiments

2. *Researchers*, who mine data to find patterns, which they use as a source of new ideas
3. *Experts*, who value proficiency in a single domain and relish opportunities to get things done
4. *Producers*, who orchestrate the activities of the network and who are the most likely members of the network to make connections across teams and groups

Innovation networks are more likely to flourish in a culture of trust and in work settings in which staff know they can safely take sensible risks to pursue excellence.

INNOVATION MILESTONES FOR A CAREER OF IMPACT

Translating innovative ideas into action and sustained success is the most difficult challenge for legacy leaders.

Sloane (2012) proposes ten actions to help healthcare executives nurture a culture of execution as well as innovation.

1. *Have a vision for change.* Legacy leaders tell aspirational stories about the vision, goals, and challenges of the organization and explain how individuals are crucial in addressing those components. They inspire staff to become passionate entrepreneurs and to find innovative routes to success.
2. *Fight the fear of change.* Innovative leaders constantly demonstrate the need for change. They replace the comfort of complacency with the hunger of ambition.
3. *Think like a venture capitalist.* Venture capitalists use a portfolio approach to balance the risk of losers with the benefits of winners.
4. *Have a dynamic suggestions program.* Leaders need not offer huge rewards. Recognition for and response to suggestions regarding change are generally more important than monetary awards. Legacy leaders acknowledge the work

Exhibit 7.1: Designing an Innovation Network

1. Connect
- Find pockets of people with right mind-sets for innovation
- Combine people with different approaches to innovation (i.e., idea generators, researchers, experts, producers)
- Ensure a mix of people with different levels of seniority and skills as well as performance
- Define as 1 network or include sub-networks devoted to specific tasks, objectives

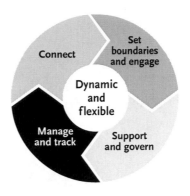

2. Set boundaries and engage
- Define role of network in meeting organization's strategic goals
- Establish network goals and objectives, as well as targets for success
- Define clear expectations
- Establish time frame and time commitment required
- Plan how to establish trust among network members and engage them quickly

3. Support and govern
- Define network's sponsorship and leadership
- Determine technology support required for network members
- Determine role of face-to-face meetings
- Define additional support as necessary (e.g., facilitators, administrative help)
- Define key knowledge and information inputs—both internal and external to network

4. Manage and track
- Define how members will be recognized for contributions
- Establish performance-management criteria based on both individual and group successes
- Establish tracking criteria
- Define timing for assessment, review and modification of network, and determine who will have these responsibilities
- Decide how new members enter network and current members leave
- Plan process to facilitate network and its impact

Source: Barsh, Capozzi, and Davidson; Exhibit 2 from "Leadership and innovation," January 2008, *McKinsey Quarterly,* www.mckinseyquarterly.com. Copyright © McKinsey & Company. Reprinted by permission.

and thought involved even when suggestions are not implemented, which can inspire new creative ideas.

5. *Break the rules.* Legacy leaders challenge complacency and encourage the lateral thinker who can create new ways to provide the goods and services that customers want.

6. *Give everyone two jobs.* Innovative leaders provide each person on their staff with two key objectives: (1) perform their current job in the most effective way possible and (2) find completely new ways to do the job.

7. *Collaborate beyond your organization.* You cannot do it all using internal resources, so look outside for other organizations with which to benchmark and partner.

8. *Welcome failure.* The innovative leader encourages a culture of experimentation. That means people must have the freedom to fail as well as succeed.

9. *Build prototypes.* Leaders should encourage staff to pilot test ideas to discover customers' reactions. A company learns far more in the real world than in the test laboratory or through focus groups.

10. *Be passionate.* A legacy leader's energy and drive translate to direction and inspiration for the entire organization. Leaders who want to inspire people to innovate, change the way they do things, and achieve extraordinary results must be passionate about what they believe in and communicate that passion every time they speak.

> **"I've been fortunate** to lead both healthcare delivery and healthcare insurance systems. In both, a leader's legacy often is not intentionally planned. It is shaped by how she or he shapes and is shaped by community leaders on our boards, and by how we shape those we invite to our management teams.
>
> While the CEO position can sometimes seem alone on a limb, the excitement comes by helping develop those around you. Expect surprises. Have a clear vision, and always pursue what you believe is the right path to achieve it.**"**
>
> **—Patrick G. Hays, FACHE**

Passion, perhaps more than any other approach, can energize the organization and promote creative and innovative thinking.

When Steve Jobs, longtime CEO of Apple, died in 2011, his death certificate listed his occupation as entrepreneur. Countless news articles described him as an icon, the modern-day equivalent of Thomas Edison or Henry Ford. No doubt he forever changed technology and the American culture; one could even argue that Jobs was the greatest innovator of our lifetime. What can we learn about innovation from Jobs? In his 2005 commencement address at Stanford University, he offered this advice:

1. Connect the dots between your past experience and your new knowledge. You cannot do this looking forward, only looking back.
2. Trust that it will work out. Have the confidence to follow your heart.
3. Find what you love, and love what you do.
4. Do not be trapped by dogma. Follow your heart and your intuition.
5. Stay hungry, and stay foolish. This was part of Jobs' formula for success.

(His complete address can be found at www.ted.com/talks/lang/en/steve_jobs_how_to_live_before_you_die.html.)

The passion for innovation and the road less traveled can guide your journey along your legacy road map. It is by leading for innovation that legacy leaders can serve as the "accelerators" described by Patricia Gabow, MD, one of the interviewed leaders featured in this book (an excerpt of her earlier quote follows).

> **❝I think great leaders act as 'accelerators' to the work and talents** of those around them. My grandfather would say '. . . If you have a gift and you don't use it, no confessor on earth can absolve you.'❞
> **—Patricia Gabow, MD**

THREE KEY ACTIONS TO HARDWIRE INNOVATION INTO YOUR LEGACY ROAD MAP

Action 1: Commit to learning about design thinking and the processes and systems for innovation evolving from centers for continuous process improvement. Examples are the Mayo Clinic Center for Innovation and the American Productivity and Quality Center (www.apqc.org).

Action 2: Expect your managers to celebrate and support sensible risk taking and a drive for continuous performance improvement among their staff, and unequivocally convey that expectation.

Action 3: Role model your personal passion for challenging the status quo and receptivity to creative ways to design programs and solve problems.

CHAPTER 8

Celebration Matters

How would you like your leadership career to be celebrated?

If you are intentional about creating your legacy, people attending your funeral will not have to wonder what your life was all about. But our interviews with the 21 healthcare leaders featured in this book remind us that it is not enough *to hope* our careers will deserve celebration; we must first celebrate the good work of those around us. Maxwell (2008, 244) shares three insights that can guide the development and use of a legacy road map that is infused with a sense of celebration:

1. Choose today the legacy you want to leave to others, at work and in your personal life.
2. Live today the legacy you want to leave. Most people don't get to choose when or how they're going to die. But they can decide how they're going to live.
3. Appreciate today the value of a good legacy. There is a great joy in taking others to places they have never been and to heights they have never dreamed possible. As a leader, you have a great opportunity to do those things.

Many leaders experience, or transmit to staff, guilt surrounding achievement of organizational or personal accomplishments. But guilt does not effectively motivate leaders or followers to fulfill bold visions. Recognition and celebration, on the other hand, are more likely to deliver sustained results and careers of impact. An authentic healthcare leader does not need to personally own the success of others; instead, he revels in their accomplishments because rewarding good behavior provides returns of sustained effort. This chapter presents tips on ways to establish a culture of celebration within healthcare organizations.

CREATING A CELEBRATION ENVIRONMENT

During recent consulting work in Eastern Europe, we discovered that every culture has useful ways to communicate insights into effective leadership; sometimes that knowledge is shared by expressing what works and what does not. To convey the need for healthcare leaders to balance positive motivation with negative sanctions, hospital managers in Eastern Europe use a powerful twist on the "carrot and stick" expression common in US management literature known as the "whip and honey" approach.

For a legacy leader, the bottom line is this: *Great management is born when recognition and celebration are added to complete the character of leaders.* Gostick and Elton (2007, 168–69) refer to this moment as "the carrot principle." It is a simple concept that emphasizes the power of recognition and reward (rather than punishment) as a positive inducement for behavior change. Unlike a fad or a trend, the carrot principle does not go out of style every few years. Gostick and Elton note that it endures and can be applied in many ways. This type of positive recognition accelerates business results along your legacy journey, amplifies the impact of every action and quickens every process, heightens your ability to see employees' achievements, sharpens your communication skills, creates cause for celebration, boosts trust between you and your employees, and improves accountability.

A 200,000-person study conducted by The Jackson Organization and reported by Gostick and Elton (2007, 168–69) confirms that leaders who achieve enhanced business results are significantly more likely to be seen by their employees as strong in the "basic four" areas of leadership:

- Goal setting
- Communication
- Trust
- Accountability

A culture of celebration magnifies these desirable skills in the leader, and when these leadership skills are present, they in turn enhance productivity in employees.

A growing body of evidence supports this notion that people perform at higher levels when they are appreciated and encouraged. Legacy leaders act on their acknowledgment that personal recognition and group celebration create the spirit and momentum that can carry a group forward even during the toughest challenges.

CELEBRATION AS CULTURE

A culture of celebration does not just happen and will not be sustained unless the leaders intentionally cultivate it. What actions do they take to harness the power of celebration?

Clarifying the Power of Celebration

Legacy leaders champion an enduring culture of celebration, not just sporadically implementing awards programs, by following Parker's (2002) steps to clarify the power of celebration in an organization.

First, legacy leaders invest in celebrations to build pride and commitment among team members. In healthcare organizations where staff are stretched thin and are expected to do more with less, pride and commitment are extraordinarily motivating factors. When healthcare team members are proud of their team and the services they produce, they generally are vested in the success of the team and work harder to achieve the team's goals.

Second, effective executives offer rewards that provide powerful motivation for staff and colleagues to explore new strategies and continuous process improvements.

Have conversations within your organization about which of these recognition or reward options might best work in your environment:

- Project management leader opportunities
- Praise
- Parking privileges
- Payments—team based or individual
- Profits
- Promotions
- Plaques
- Pats on the back
- Pizza
- Prizes

The healthcare leaders we interviewed for this book indicated that most individuals learn the positive and negative reactions for good and bad behaviors early in life. By celebrating accomplishments, leaders encourage their team members to continue the behaviors being celebrated.

Third, they frame celebration as a support mechanism for the growth of a healthy team culture. When a team celebrates a success, the environment of the team becomes or remains positive.

A thank-you note is an effective way to demonstrate recognition, appreciation, and encouragement. Successful healthcare leaders tap the power of a hand-written personal thank you in this digital age wherein the quick and easy e-mail may seem an impersonal "cut and paste." Superficial communication may seem insincere and prove counterproductive, while the hand-written note demonstrates that the leader cares enough about staff's efforts to take the time to personally acknowledge them.

Embracing Celebration as Both a Process and an Event

The atmosphere of effective celebration events is informal and upbeat. Celebrations can promote team cohesion and enhance member relationships in a nonformal, nonthreatening way. Legacy leaders continuously establish opportunities for celebration.

Some years ago, a hospital system leader thanked one of her staff members in a unique way. She not only thanked him in front of his coworkers for a job done well and on time but sent a personalized letter to his wife and another to his mother noting how proud they must be to have such an exemplary husband and son. Not only did those two women reinforce the celebrations after hours, but the manager felt a positive glow of pride for weeks after the event. Such a gift of celebration is remembered and contributes to her lasting legacy as an effective leader.

THE ROLE OF EMOTIONAL INTELLIGENCE IN EMBRACING CELEBRATION

To fulfill the celebration leg of the legacy road map, leaders should develop high emotional intelligence (EQ). As introduced in Chapter 2, EQ is related to but distinct from cognitive intelligence, measured by the intelligence quotient, or IQ. EQ is at the root of our ability to unravel social complexities by perceiving, generating, and managing emotions in ourselves and others. Sometimes referred to as "street smarts" or "common sense," EQ embodies skills required to understand and manage our interior emotional lives and to negotiate the shoals of social interactions. Emotionally intelligent leaders communicate effectively, form strong relationships, and create powerful coping strategies at work and in their personal lives. They are also more likely to live and leave positive legacies.

Stein and colleagues (2009) found that celebrating staff members' demonstrations of EQ in terms of five core factors—perceiving, managing, decision making, achieving, and influencing—maximizes emotional and social functioning. Legacy leaders intentionally cultivate a culture of celebration and thereby nourish all of these factors. Exhibit 8.1 illustrates this relationship.

Perceiving and managing are shown in the middle of the exhibit because these two factors are central to effectively using EQ. A leader who cannot perceive and manage emotions appropriately will have difficulty with the remaining three factors. Although decision making, achieving, and influencing are shown in the model in a linear fashion, these factors are all used at varying times when a leader applies EQ.

Because legacy leaders are emotionally intelligent, they are celebration smart as well. Celebration and recognition efforts ring hollow if they are presented in an insincere manner or awarded on the basis of sloppy performance targets or disorganized processes.

Exhibit 8.1: Emotional Intelligence Skills Assessment (EISA)

PERCEIVING
The ability to accurately recognize, attend to, and understand emotion.

DECISION MAKING
The appropriate application of emotion to manage change and solve problems

ACHIEVING
The ability to generate the necessary emotions to self-motivate in the pursuit of realistic and meaningful objectives.

INFLUENCING
The ability to recognize, manage, and evoke emotion within oneself and others to promote change

MANAGING
The ability to effectively manage, control, and express emotions.

Source: "Emotional Intelligence Skills Assessment (EISA)," by Steven J. Stein, Derek Mann, Peter Papadogiannis, and Wendy Gordon. Copyright © 2009 John Wiley & Sons, Inc. Reproduced with permission of John Wiley & Sons, Inc.

Leaders with high EQ use the following three principles to guide the cultivation of a celebration culture:

1. They clearly communicate that they value the achievement of stretch performance goals (many legacy leaders now use the balanced scorecard framework with a measurable target for quality, service volumes, pride, financial vitality, and continuous improvement).
2. They mutually set, rigorously monitor, and transparently report goals, plans, and progress for each manager and organizational unit.
3. They openly recognize and celebrate progress, taking particular care to provide praise in public and reprimand, if necessary, in private.

Recognition and reward initiatives can be implemented in all types of health systems: public and private, wealthy and poor.

FORMS OF PERFORMANCE PRAISE

During a recent exercise at the International Health Leadership Program at Cambridge University, we asked public-sector hospital leaders from 20 countries to define ways to show appreciation for work well done. Even in civil service settings, with little extra cash for incentives or merit pay, several forms of performance praise were suggested, including the following:

- Praise as close to the time and place of the good work as possible.
- Offer whatever incentives for peak performance the civil service structures allow, such as better parking, office accommodations, clerical staff access to special training programs, and educational travel.
- Conduct visible award and recognition programs for staff, and invite awardees' families to see and hear the praise from bosses and colleagues.

- Offer additional days off with pay.
- Allow staff to perform or lead special projects or studies seen as important to the overall goals of the organization (the prestige of being selected to make a difference is itself rewarding).
- Allow job rotation as a way to increase the potential for future promotions and advancements.
- Invite leaders who perform well to social events, such as dinners with senior and respected leaders.
- Take an interest in staff's life and career trends or patterns on an individual level. Demonstrate that interest in a sincere manner.
- Nominate high performers for local, regional, national, and international award programs. If your organization does not have the funds for a special award, others might. Even the act of the nomination is a reward that brings benefit to the organization as well as the individual.
- In a very open and transparent process, assign point values that high performers may earn toward receiving reasonable donated gifts from suppliers.
- Negotiate a bundle of special leave packages with central civil service that can be used for teams that exceed expectations for the patients, community, or agency.
- Publish a photo book of the high performers on the organization's website or as a hard-copy insert to a publication each quarter for colleagues, family, and neighbors to view.
- Institute department-wide incentives to earn better equipment, office furniture, access to education programs, or cash bonuses for exceeding targets.
- Offer flexible hours or work prerogatives to high achievers.
- Recognize high performers where most of the work is done—on the front line—with a pat on the back in front of their colleagues.
- Hand out plaques recognizing great work, creative ideas, or innovative process improvements.

- Offer vouchers for dinners, entertainment, travel, food packages, sports equipment, books, publications, and so forth to those who exceed goals.
- Create opportunities every quarter for staff to work in another job for cross-education and training development, or just for positive change of pace or for fun.
- Post pictures of high performers in public areas to celebrate their great work and positive attitudes.
- Reward the staff of high-achieving departments with afternoon neck massages for a month.
- Empower staff to engage in shared decision making. This empowerment carries its own incentive and allows more people to have a stake in their destiny.
- Fire bad managers, or move them to a more suitable position, if they do not demonstrate good role-modeling behavior.
- Listen, or listen better, to workers about how their work and processes could be improved. Once you have acknowledged their observations, ask them how you can be more effective as a leader.

Legacy leaders influence those around them with praise as well as pay. Healthcare leaders would do well to review how they balance sincere praise with creative incentive pay.

CELEBRATION AND A LEGACY OF LEADERSHIP

Leaders who intentionally develop and nurture organizational cultures with high performance expectations and who creatively celebrate excellent performance also embody many of the skills discussed throughout this book, such as mentoring; investing in manager and team development; being aware of the value of eclectic teams characterized by diversity in age, gender, ethnicity, and work experience; being visionary; and showing support for a passionate pursuit of innovation.

To begin building a legacy road map that features a culture of celebration, consider Oden's (2009) "distinguished dozen" observations:

1. Legacy leaders are remembered for their interpersonal skills, EQ, and ability to quickly transform a group into a vision-driven team.
2. People do not remember the titles of legacy leaders as much as they remember those leaders' credibility, influence, compassion, understanding, patience, and integrity.
3. Legacy leaders are courageous. They are willing to stand for what is right and to take risks with a quiet tenacity. They also are willing to "go against the flow" to ensure that the highest standards are maintained.
4. Legacy leaders look inward before acting outward. They know their motivations, vulnerabilities, and triggers for negative emotions. They are authentic and teachable.
5. Legacy leaders know how and when to be quiet. They ask questions and take the time to research and discover all the details before forming an opinion or taking action.
6. Legacy leaders are teachers. They remember that everyone is in a state of growth. They know that each day offers opportunities for continuous improvement, not perfection, and they encourage those they lead to strive for learning.
7. Legacy leaders are approachable. They create safe environments into which others know they can bring concerns or new ideas.
8. Legacy leaders know how to balance managing by influence and managing by authority.
9. Legacy leaders are empowering. They ensure the success of those around them. They plan for and train their successors.

They inspire others to stretch and grow through support and positioning for success.

10. Legacy leaders do not build more followers; they build more leaders.

11. Legacy leaders are visionary. They visualize tomorrow's possibilities, see the organization's potential, and break down the steps to allow their staff the opportunity to experience small successes on their journey to vision attainment.

12. Legacy leaders set an example of excellence, not perfection.

To successfully apply these initiatives across their organizations, legacy leaders listen carefully to the ideas and heed the wisdom of their staff, viewing them as colleagues and partners in a journey to high performance. Invite ideas from staff about topics from performance goals to obstacles inhibiting goal achievement to how to distribute awards and hold celebrations.

THREE KEY ACTIONS TO HARDWIRE CELEBRATION INTO YOUR LEGACY ROAD MAP

Action 1: Subscribe to three e-newsletters that push fresh ideas and insights to your e-mail. Scan news about advances in talent management regarding employee- and team-based recognition and rewards.

Action 2: With your senior leadership team, develop an enhanced approach to recognition and reward programming for frontline and middle managers that includes
- an assessment to determine the degree of receptivity to and trust in a new culture of recognition and rewards for enhanced care and departmental performance,

- a forum for staff to safely share their views on criteria and processes for credible celebration events and rewards, and
- board-level commitment for a sustainable budget to support ongoing celebration.

Action 3: Make a meaningful effort to champion and role model a spirit of celebration for your direct reports and colleagues.

PART III

Your Career Life Cycle

CHAPTER 9

Encore Performance

A LEADER'S PERSONAL and professional impact extends well beyond the day one retires. Once the executive is no longer "held hostage" by the job and the need to make a living, he can live a life that significantly affects the field, the profession, and the community in ways that were not possible on the job.

The retirement years afford leaders the time for reflection and self-examination and the opportunity to make up for the "unexamined life." Retirement is often the signal event that prompts a serious accounting of one's personal and professional life. What, if any, meaningful contribution has been made, and perhaps just as importantly, what has been learned that should be shared? In this context, *to retire* should be an action verb, as retirement is one's second chance to enhance or establish a memorable legacy.

However, as indicated earlier in the book, many healthcare leaders wait too long to plan for their retirement. We often talk to leaders as they are about to retire, and we find they have no clue how to thrive in their next 10 to 20 years. Leaders with 30-year careers spent guiding multimillion-dollar enterprises by following well-defined plans tend to drift into their first decade of retirement. In this chapter, we aim to redefine and invigorate the concept of retirement as part of your legacy road map.

> **"Retired healthcare** leaders need to maintain a holistic approach to life and pay attention to mind, body, and spirit. There will be opportunity and time to connect with family and consider their legacy."
>
> —John G. King, LFACHE

REINVENTING RETIREMENT

Those retiring in the current decade will not experience the retirement of their grandfathers—or of their fathers. First, Andrew Weil, MD, (2005, 6) observes that "we won't age the way our parents and grandparents did." We have access to better healthcare, more knowledge about the prevention of age-related disease, better access to healthy food, and products and services available to accommodate us as we age; we understand the importance of physical fitness, exercise, and stress management; and we know the hazards of smoking and other addictive behaviors.

Second, this is the boomer generation, and its members "will not go quietly into retirement." Rosabeth Moss Kanter, as quoted by Lloyd (2009, 7, 10), predicts that "having been told from birth about their own significance, they aren't going to feel less significant simply because they have hit a career ceiling called retirement age." This is the generation that lays claim to the sexual revolution, Vietnam War protests, landmark civil rights legislation, and free love, so as Moss Kanter says, "they naturally feel like world changers."

Freedman (2007, 3) agrees, adding that "Longevity, demography, human development, generational experience, fiscal imperatives, labor market dictates, and historical moment combined [may] lead boomers to contribute longer and to use their education and experience . . . to [add] deeper meaning . . . and broader

> "Retirement should be a positive transition. Contemplation, reading, and research about transitions [are] very helpful prior to retirement. Don't assume your retirement life will be business as usual. You must develop a vision for this next chapter of your life because your life will be very different."
>
> **—Patrick G. Hays, FACHE**

> "Don't wait until you retire to think about how you want to spend this next stage of life. Don't be totally involved with work—and then retire the next day. You need to start early to develop your interests—even while you're working. The transition is more dramatic than you think."
>
> **—Ed Dahlberg, LFACHE**

social purposes" to the retirement experience. He further predicts that boomers "will swap income for impact" (Freedman 2007, 5–6). In the type of scenario laid out by Moss Kanter and Freedman, the boomer legacy may be to change the way that the world thinks about the purpose of work and how it defines success (Bauer-Maglin and Radosh 2003, 4). The boomers who came of age in the 1960s left college determined to create a better world and got sidetracked. Now they have a second chance, and they are better equipped than previous generations of retirees to be change agents because they are more energetic, politically astute, and financially secure.

Third, as Laura Carstensen (2001) says in her *New York Times* article "On the Brink of a Brand-New Old Age," we need to have a new conversation about retirement that involves more than prescription drug benefits and Social Security eligibility. As Satchel Paige, legendary baseball player, once mused, "How old would you be if you didn't know how old you was?" The very definition of retirement needs reexamination. A *new* image for retirement is beginning to take shape. It has begun to be seen as an opportunity for adventure, encore work, community service, artistic achievement, and legacy building.

THE THIRD AGE

Sadler (2000) tells us that the course of life can be divided into four ages. The first age is for learning, the second for work, the third for living, and the fourth for aging. He says the "vast, scarcely known region in the middle of our lives constitutes the third age, a new frontier with tremendous potential for growth" and claims these "additional years that we can expect to extend our lives are like hitting the lottery" (Sadler 2000). Indeed, for many of us it will be an additional 30 years.

The question of how we will spend this time looms. As we age, we become increasingly aware that our time in the here and now is finite. Retirement represents a "final gift of time to be used authentically and with good intent" (Bauer-Maglin and Radosh 2003, 4). For many of us, success in our careers has often been viewed as our "legacy," but career success can also have a dark side. Some people "succeed in careers but lose in life"; in retirement, those who lose in life have a chance to transform the rest of their time to a richer, more vibrant, and more meaningful life than we ever imagined. The third age can be the surprise opportunity to establish or enhance one's legacy (Sadler 2000).

Another factor is that we have traditionally been identified by what we do rather than by who we are. As Sadler (2000, 8) puts it, more than a few professionals have a strikingly impoverished sense of self. They have not taken the time to examine who they are or to develop interests or relationships outside of work.

> **"I've always lived my life knowing there would be another chapter. I'm a violinist, and my goal in my retirement from healthcare is to play in an orchestra. I know that I need a plan to prepare for this."**
>
> **—Nancy M. Schlichting**

However, Freedman (2007) says we are beginning to see a cultural shift as well as an economic shift in our society. He predicts a movement from materialism into more community work, with a desire of many entering this third age "to better care for, sustain and promote the well-being of our society and the earth."

Rather than decline, aging can bring "depth and richness of experience, complexity of being, serenity, wisdom, and its own kind of power and grace"; because aging reminds us of our mortality, it can be a primary stimulus to spiritual awakening and growth (Weil 2005). What an incredible opportunity to create one's own epitaph.

WHAT WORK GIVES US

What does work do for us besides pay the bills? Work provides a sense of direction and a reason to get up in the morning. It often becomes our very identity.

Work also is our connection with people. It provides us with a network of friends and colleagues in a social setting. These connections and this sense of purpose contribute to positive self-esteem and a sense of well-being we hope to carry throughout our careers. In fact, their absence can lead to mental and physical deterioration, according to Freedman (2007, 81).

> "When I thought about retirement, I decided that I wanted to make an impact but on a much smaller scale. I wanted to be able to see the difference I was making. I think this may be a common desire among retiring executives."
> —Patrick G. Hays, FACHE

Does this mean one should continue working well past retirement age at a job one knows and performs well? That is not the suggestion here. Many of us, especially in a beleaguered industry like healthcare, reach a point where our job is no longer challenging, it has become too challenging, or it is no longer appealing. Maybe we are bored, are frustrated, or just need a change of pace. Or maybe we have more compelling things we would like to do. Retirement provides the freedom to live your life the way you wish, to do the things you have always wanted to do but have never had the time to act on.

So while working into retirement age provides benefits for both society (older workers lend their experience and knowledge to solving future labor shortages) and the workers themselves (from the supplemental income and daily structure), we need to rethink work and how we define it to make it meaningful as we embrace the third age. Business writer Charles Handy suggests that we

> "Unfortunately, many of us do not know 'how to let go' once we have retired. We need to get the message out there that one needs to prepare and to reinvent oneself for this inevitable transition."
> —Donald C. Wegmiller, FACHE

construct an "enlarged work portfolio" in which we include different kinds of work: paid work, volunteer work, home work, religious work, political work, grandparenting, environmental work, personal development, health promotion, fun work, and learning (Sadler 2000, 100–101). This portfolio can be kept current with retirement activities and serve as one's authentic curriculum vita. As a whole, the portfolio should reflect the type of life that you find rewarding.

In redefining work, we are redefining success as well. Rather than income and status as the metrics, intrinsic rewards of living a meaningful life, self-development, and service to others are our measures. In choosing work aimed at making a better world, this generation of retirees could be redefining success for all of society. Could there possibly be a better legacy than that?

GET READY, GET SET, GO!

Retirement is a life transition that requires serious long-term planning and self-assessment. Most people define retirement planning strictly in financial terms and fail to consider the emotional and social adjustments that come with it. In fact, the majority of people spend more time planning a two-week vacation than they do their retirement; the average American spends 90,000 hours working toward retirement and fewer than 10 hours planning for it (Cullinane and Fitzgerald 2007, xi). To avoid this trend, try planning for your retirement the way you plan for your organization—and start early. Our aim is to help you stimulate thoughtful reflection and self-discovery and to motivate you to develop a lifestyle vision that maximizes your potential for a fulfilling, productive, and rewarding next stage of life.

The Health Factor

Before we proceed, however, we pause to remind you of the impact your health has on your third-age years. Take charge of your health early on to avoid painful, disruptive, and expensive chronic conditions later. Staying healthy means you will shell out less for medical care *and* reduce a major threat to your financial security in retirement.

Perhaps more relevant, ill health may prevent you from leading the active, participatory future life you have planned. Well-being during this portion of our lives requires more discipline than at any previous point in life, but the rewards are greater. By paying attention to our health, we can dramatically change the way we age for the better, as caring well for our bodies improves intellectual and emotional functions and helps us to remain vital, healthy, and independent members of society (Sadler 2000, 163–64).

In good health, then, we are prepared to confidently move forward to build or enhance a legacy that those we care about can be proud of.

> **It can be difficult for CEOs to no longer have staff to do their** bidding. Newly retired executives must be realistic about what they can do by themselves and when they may need to affiliate with an organization.
>
> It is important that retired healthcare leaders be engaged in something that has meaning and keeps their intellect sharp. Retired healthcare executives need to stay flexible. Plans may be redirected.
>
> —John G. King, LFACHE

ENCORE CAREERS

A study by Merrill Lynch cited by Lloyd (2009, 6–10) found that two-thirds of Americans say they will work in some kind of job for pay during retirement (the persistence of the current economic downturn may have increased that number). Despite some obvious disadvantages, working later into life can score a "financial hat trick," with more years to save, fewer years to live off your savings, and the ability to draw larger Social Security payments. Add healthcare coverage to that equation, and working can be an attractive option.

The prospect of more retirement-age persons in the workplace is good news. Business magazines and think tanks warn of skilled labor deficits and an alarming experience drain in the near future. The nonprofit sector reports that aging senior managers are creating a leadership deficit that will require at least 1 million managers in the next ten years to reverse (Freedman 2007, 78). The MetLife Foundation and Civic Ventures, a think tank working on issues concerning baby boomers, work, and social purpose, reports that by 2018, at least 5 million jobs could be vacant in the United States, nearly half of them social-sector jobs in education, healthcare, government, and nonprofit organizations (Bluestone and Melnik 2010). Civic Ventures CEO Marc Freedman testified before the US Senate Finance Committee on July 15, 2010, with the message that "it's time to provide incentives to help millions more people find encore careers that provide continued income, personal meaning and social impact."

We discuss three examples of activities to help you choose the type of encore career you might want to pursue: sharing your knowledge, making a difference through volunteering, and grandparenting.

> **"In this next chapter of my life, I would like to work in the arts—** I would like to work in ways where I can see the connection to helping people.**"**
>
> **—Nancy M. Schlichting**

Sharing Your Knowledge

"Sharing your knowledge is the way to achieve immortality," notes the Dalai Lama. It is no accident that many retired healthcare professionals pursue writing, teaching, consulting, and governing board service, areas in which they have valuable lessons to share and the motivation to give back to the profession. The intrinsic rewards of giving back to the field may far outweigh any professional or monetary gains. Sharing may be seen as especially important in this stage of life because some healthcare professionals may have spent years in a competitive, corporate environment where sharing was frowned upon (Sadler 2000, 61). The focus in the encore career is on having an impact, not on career advancement (Weiss 2005, 4). The thoughtful reflection and self-discovery we advocate earlier in this book allows you to take stock of your life, the wisdom you have gained, and the lessons you have learned. It may come as a surprise that you have so much of value to share.

Consulting once was almost a stereotypical retirement job. However, surveys now show that the first choice of work in retirement among retiring healthcare executives is teaching (Freedman 2007, 23). Students are eager to learn from experienced professionals, and those professionals now serving as faculty enjoy the enthusiasm of students benefiting from their knowledge. An alternative to teaching, or a complementary side activity, is career counseling, and either occupation may develop into mentoring of young professionals that extends well beyond the classroom.

MAKING A DIFFERENCE THROUGH VOLUNTEERING

Volunteering to work in political, religious, environmental, or charitable organizations that have real social impact can fill one's life with purpose and satisfaction. Bringing a lifetime of experience and skills to worthwhile organizations is often a meaningful contribution for the retirement-age executive. Communities, institutions, and the environment benefit from volunteer participation, leading to success of an organizational mission that otherwise might be out of reach.

> **"Retire like you** mean it! You're not letting go—you're moving on to new opportunities, new adventures.**"**
> —**Ed Dahlberg**, LFACHE

Working on a political campaign allows you to promote your personal political agenda. Many faith-based initiatives that support social ministries offer volunteer opportunities. Public school districts throughout the United States need teaching assistants, tutors, and volunteers in all aspects of their programs. Charities that promote health and research are always clamoring for volunteers. In short, the meaningful volunteer opportunity of your choice is most likely only a telephone call away.

Volunteer activity can bring significant value to the recipient organization, especially during an economic downturn when many nonprofit organizations suffer staffing shortages, reduced government funding of social welfare programs, and diminished donor giving. Programs threatened with extinction may see volunteers as their salvation. In times of such need, volunteers may quickly witness the results of their labors, making their work even more gratifying, better recognized, and more appreciated.

If you feel you need to prepare for such an encore role, consider seeking to join a program that facilitates learning for retiring executives. For example, Moss Kanter is working with others at Harvard University to develop advanced leadership schools to teach retirement-age leaders skills they can apply to improving their community, their region, and the world. The concept redefines later life and the role of higher education in preparing retired workers to be community leaders and to use their experience for the social good.

Another program, the Impact Awards, was created by AARP to honor people who have improved the world we live in. One past honoree is Richard Gere, a well-known actor and humanitarian who really did not have to do anything to preserve his place in history. But he is quoted as saying, "A few years ago I said, 'Look, I have so many years left, maybe, to accomplish something of value.'" He created Healing the Divide, a public charity dedicated to helping communities in Asia, the Middle East, and the United States tackle pressing social and cultural issues. Few, if any, of us have Gere's resources, but we will have time, energy, and expertise to give in ways that will make an impact, and along the way help to build our legacy.

Grandparenting in the Twenty-first Century

Grandparenting now is very different from grandparenting in the past, when grandmothers wore aprons and baked cookies and grandfathers wore sweaters and smoked pipes and they lived just over the river and through the woods. Today's grandparents may live near or far from their grandchildren, and they will have varying levels of interest and responsibility in the lives of their grandchildren. It is generally accepted that today's grandparents are typically healthier, wealthier, and better educated than the grandparents of the past. Overall, they will live longer than any previous generation of grandparents and thus will have the opportunity to be grandparents for a much longer period of time.

Today's grandchildren are very different, as well. As a group, they are smarter, more technologically advanced, busier, and more sophisticated than grandchildren of the past. In some ways, they are more independent and worldly as a result of facing issues and stressors that were unknown to the children and adolescents of previous generations. In other ways, they are more dependent on adults because they need help navigating the sometimes murky waters of this formative period of their lives.

The roles and responsibilities of grandparents can be as diverse as the imagination. Some grandparents may take on the role of caregiver—part time or more often, depending on circumstance and choice. Wisdom about child development and proper discipline has been gained through experience, past mistakes, and the determination not to repeat them. Other grandparents may serve as teachers, nurturing learning and providing support and encouragement for academic achievement. Still others may support the efforts of their grandchildren in sports or the arts. By virtue of their position in the family, grandparents serve as powerful role models who help to set the standards and values for morally acceptable behaviors.

Grandparents also serve the transitional role of helping bridge the generations, which typically span 100 years or more of family history. In this regard, grandparents can be seen as the great custodians of time and as a connection to infinity (Exhibit 9.1). Family history and traditions are kept alive and passed on to future generations through stories, photographs, family Bibles, baptismal records, school certificates, diplomas, marriage certificates, immigration papers, passports, and the like. Grandchildren strengthen a retiree's sense of family continuity and become their "emissaries to the future" (Weiss 2005, 161).

Few dispute the unique emotional bond that exists between grandparents and their grandchildren. Modern technology makes it easier for the disparate generations to stay connected today. Even great geographic distances can be easily spanned with Skype,

Exhibit 9.1: Grandparents as the Fulcrum of the Family

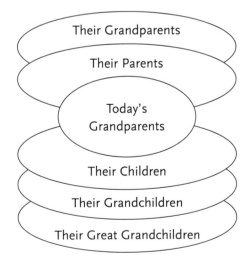

Facebook, e-mail, and the more conventional telephone (audio) and DVD (video) recordings. Grandchildren often feel more comfortable seeking advice and counsel from grandparents, with whom they often have a bond built on unconditional love.

Those of us who are fortunate to live long enough to become grandparents should consider this longevity a gift—one that comes with responsibilities and rewards. If you believe we have an obligation to give back to society, what better way to do so than to help future generations to make society a better place? The rewards are significant: a purpose for living one's life, enjoyment, companionship, activity, and a passion for living that contributes to good health and a sense of well-being. Some years ago, when I asked my father if he believed in reincarnation, he said, "I believe our immortality rests within our grandchildren, so grandparents should pay careful attention to the nurturing of these young souls."

The need and the opportunity exist for grandparents to make a significant and meaningful contribution to their families and to society. In doing so, they may leave a legacy built on the simplicity of love. They may also find that choosing to do so brings a renewed joie de vivre.

DISPELLING THE MYTHS ABOUT RETIREMENT

If you are to legitimately build on your legacy in retirement and have an impact on your profession or your community, you must learn to navigate the myths that can get in your way.

The first surrounds the stereotypes associated with aging and retirement as a period of nothing more than decline. Once we retire, we become that invisible segment of the population that is perceived as crowding our healthcare system, driving up healthcare costs, and bankrupting future generations of Americans through Medicare and Social Security; it is only a matter of time before we become a burden to our families as well as to society. We can fight this myth by the way we live our lives and by ridding our conversations of humor based on menopause, Alzheimer's disease, and other consequences of aging, which reinforce these stereotypes.

The second myth is that retirement is automatically a period of decline. Instead, it is being seen more and more as a period of potential new growth. The workplace is being redefined to embrace encore careers and retirement-age workers' significant contributions to the community, the environment, and the planet. Success in our careers is being redefined as success in life. Rather than fear, our sense of our own mortality has become a motivation to build a legacy that anyone can be proud of.

The third myth about retirement is that we can fight aging. According to Weil (2005, 6), to deny aging and to think we can fight it is counterproductive; rather than seek Botox and Viagra, he says, our goal should be to "live as long as possible and as well as possible, then have a rapid decline at the end of life." Meeting that goal requires that we work at being as healthy, engaged, and productive as possible well into our retirement.

Finally, the most dangerous myth of retirement is that "you can and should put off what is really important in your life now—because someday if you save enough money, you'll get to do what you really want to do, give and be" (Bach 2005, 310). If you buy into this way of thinking, you will miss out on your whole life.

Henry James once said, "The great use of life is to spend it for something that will outlast us." You are the architect of the lifelong construction of your legacy. You are building a career of impact as you are building your life. Your legacy does not begin in your retirement and it does not end when you retire. The impact you make is an evolutionary process that ends only when you decide.

> **"Healthcare leaders contemplating retirement would be wise to** consider the advice of philosopher Joseph Campbell: 'Follow your bliss and the universe will open doors for you where there were only walls.'"
>
> **—John G. King, LFACHE**

THREE KEY ACTIONS TO HARDWIRE ENCORE PERFORMANCE INTO YOUR LEGACY ROAD MAP

Action 1: Reflect now on how you may wish to live the third age of your life's journey. What more will you want to accomplish? With family? With community? What work might you wish to engage in and how might you prepare for it? Begin to expand your SMART (specific, measurable, attainable, realistic, and timely) career goals to include your retirement years.

Action 2: Commit now to a personal health and fitness program that will help inoculate you against expensive, inconvenient, and painful chronic disease and disability in the future.

Action 3: Begin to gather information on how to live a rich and rewarding retirement by reading books and articles by authorities on the subject and by seeking the advice of retired healthcare executives. What has their experience taught them? What would they do differently in these pre-retirement years?

CHAPTER 10

Conclusion: Map Your Journey

CONSULTANTS, EDUCATORS, RESEARCHERS, and our 21 healthcare executives suggest it is never too late to plan your legacy journey, but the earlier, the better. Most of the leaders interviewed for this book indicated that while they rarely worried about a legacy in their early years, they saw the value of intentionally developing those around them for organizational and personal advancement.

MAP YOUR JOURNEY

"May you live in interesting times." When Frederic Coudert referenced this Chinese proverb (or "curse") in 1939 at the Proceedings of the Academy of Political Science, he followed it with, "No age has been more fraught with insecurity than our present time." The same could be said for this decade. Legacy leaders recognize the capricious nature of our careers and deal effectively with uncertainty, scarcity, and change.

Many of society's institutions—religion, education, and government, to name a few—suffer from a crisis of public confidence and a leadership void, and healthcare is not exempt. A sea change in leadership is occurring in the field, with thousands of executives moving through transitions in a time of landmark legislation, globalization, and general uncertainty for our nation's healthcare system. The healthcare field finds itself and its leaders in uncharted waters. In this challenging era, there is a premium on excellent leaders who help organizations and staff navigate these changes and in the process create a career of impact. Considering that healthcare is the largest segment of the US economy, we have an obligation to help develop new leaders who can span boundaries to better serve both our industry and our society.

This text was written to encourage and motivate healthcare leaders to think beyond the pressing day-to-day challenges of their organizations and to plan and live careers that unleash the performance of colleagues, organizations, and communities. It was written for those who wish to create a career of impact and, in so doing, leave a meaningful legacy to their organizations, their industry, and their families. Along this path, one must be intentional about developing self-awareness, building essential mentoring skills, and enhancing the character attributes that produce leaders who make a difference.

Seven building blocks are essential for mapping a career of impact. We have explored each of these key markers as essential elements to the leadership journey. Our discussion has explored how to develop these leadership competencies and how to put them to work within one's organization and one's personal and professional life. Focused examination of these competencies was intended to challenge readers to assess their leadership skills and to develop and promote leadership skills in themselves and those around them in ways that help ensure that *their* careers make a difference as well. A review of these competencies is offered here to guide the mapping of your journey for a career of impact.

> **"A leader's effectiveness can be enhanced by people at all levels of** the organization, especially those on the front lines. Changing the culture to empower the talents of individuals and teams on the front lines is an essential component of great leadership. Earning followers comes from showing respect to all those who directly serve the organization's mission.**"**
>
> **—William C. Schoenhard, FACHE**

Building Block 1: Self-Reflection and Awareness

A great leader is self-aware; has, over the course of a career, developed the ability to distill accumulated wisdom from what has been learned; and has learned how to effectively share these insights with others. Great leaders may have many character traits, but an essential trait is to be authentic to oneself. The key to developing these skills begins early in a career. Legacy leaders know how to recognize it, develop it, and nurture it throughout their healthcare organizations.

Building Block 2: Integrity and Character

Physicians and employees in healthcare organizations are hungry to work with leaders who inspire and challenge them to achieve high levels of performance in an era of rapid change that calls for more accountable results. Character and integrity are the cornerstones of great leadership. Leadership failures are often failures of character. Strength of character requires discipline and progressive reinforcement. Advances in technology, the labyrinth of healthcare financing, healthcare reform, complex business transactions, consumer expectations, public scrutiny, legislative requirements, and the proliferation of socioeconomically induced health problems are just some of the issues that significantly increase the complexity of healthcare management. Legacy leaders frequently find themselves in uncharted waters where the ethical rules may be unclear. We have examined strategies and recommended steps to foster personal integrity and ethical conduct and support these competencies in staff throughout the organization.

We add one more component: leaving a legacy of "non-material gifts: the values and life lessons that you wish to leave to others" by writing an ethical will (Weil 2005, 288–90). Historically, ethical wills have been a part of Hindu, Zen, and Jewish traditions, but they are making a comeback in modern times because they provide an opportunity to make sense of one's life. Writing an ethical will can clarify how you want to live out the rest of your life; it can also function as the spiritual legacy that you share with your family or others important to you.

Building Block 3: Visioning—The Long View

A vision is a clear description of the desired future state of being, whether applied to organizations or individuals. Healthcare leaders who strive for a career of impact must cultivate a desired vision for their personal career as well as for their organization. Impact leaders embrace a vision that defines how both their organizations and their careers will look and behave in the future. When leaders engage their staff and colleagues to develop, embrace, and work intentionally to achieve their organizational vision—and help these colleagues and staff to understand and own that vision—staff and colleagues are more likely to work harder to achieve it. And so it is with one's personal vision. The leader's work to clarify a bold vision for a career of impact improves the probability of experiencing such a career.

Building Block 4: Mentoring and Leadership Development

Mentoring is not easy. There is both an art and a science to good mentoring. Effective mentoring is formal, intentional, and disciplined. The mentors must be willing to care about and listen to their mentees, show vulnerability, and provide opportunities for growth for a future generation of leaders. We have explored the obligations, commitment, responsibilities, obstacles, and traits inherent in leaders as effective mentors, and the powerful advantages that may accrue to both mentor and protégé. While we encourage active leaders in the field to be mentors, mentoring can be especially rewarding to retired executives and those they mentor. Protégés benefit from the increased availability of the retired mentor while the mentor benefits from continued affiliation with the field.

Building Block 5: Managing Diversity

Healthcare leaders can no longer afford to think of diversity only in terms of race and gender. Diversity that also encompasses cultural, generational, geographic, ethnic, and religious values requires different leadership skills. Further complicating the work environment is the emergence of a workforce of multidisciplinary professionals who may operate under dual lines of authority and an organization that serves myriad stakeholders with vested and sometimes opposing interests. The most critical challenge facing healthcare leaders today is to ensure that the multicultural patient population receives safe and culturally competent care. We have examined leadership issues surrounding these diverse groups and defined strategies to navigate these sometimes unfamiliar and murky waters.

> **"Leaders come in all shapes** and sizes; you do not need to be a CEO to have success as a . . . leader. Developing and supporting those around you to make a difference is key. Your contribution is also more likely if you have a deliberate plan to guide your career's development."
>
> —**Donald C. Wegmiller**, FACHE

Building Block 6: Leading Innovation

Health sector organizations must continually reinvent and improve their performance. Stakeholder demands for superior healthcare and value require continuous analysis and reflection about one's organizational strengths, weaknesses, opportunities, and threats. One's career requires this same analysis, leading to innovation in both. Leaders must master and champion innovation. Leading innovation requires visionary purpose and goals. To achieve successful outcomes, it is imperative to create a vital, sustainable organization. Colleagues are looking to healthcare leaders to champion fresh ways of looking at change and challenge. We have illustrated key points in the development of a personal road map, revealing strategies for innovation that drive improved service and performance. We have shown how to frame questions differently and address challenges through a fresh perspective.

Building Block 7: Celebration Matters

Many leaders experience, or transmit to staff, guilt surrounding organizational or personal accomplishments. But guilt does little to effectively motivate followers or achieve bold visions. Recognition and celebration, on the other hand, deliver sustained results and careers of impact. An authentic healthcare leader is not one who steals from the success of others but who revels in the success of others. Powerful leaders know that rewarding good behavior sustains a return of effort, and they have learned to celebrate the success of those around them. We have presented tips on ways to establish a culture of celebration within healthcare organizations.

ENCORE PERFORMANCE

The retirement years afford the time for reflection, the space for self-examination, and the opportunity to make up for the "unexamined life." Retirement may be the capstone career transition whereby meaningful contributions can be shared. In today's environment, *retire* is an action verb, and retirement must be seen as one's second chance to establish or enhance a memorable legacy.

One's personal and professional impact extends well beyond the day one formally retires. Once the executive is no longer "held hostage" by the job and the need to make a living, he or she can lead a life that has significant impact on the field, the profession, and the community. It is no accident that many retired professionals pursue writing, teaching, consulting, and governing board service, as they have valuable lessons to share and the motivation to serve. Planning for encore employment, meaningful volunteer work, and family and community contributions was explored.

Healthcare professionals know that networking is essential to career development. A network of colleagues to help with a job search, serve as a reference, or share advice when we are dealing with thorny issues has become indispensable. But Lloyd (2009, 37) tells us that networking is "the Super Glue of retirement years" and that, in retirement, networking is about who we can help. This kind of networking fosters a sense of connection that we no longer get from our jobs and provides us with a unique opportunity to play a special role in preparing the next generation to make their contributions.

CONCLUSION

This text has focused on both job effectiveness and career effectiveness and has sought to bridge the two in ways that strengthen both. It explores how to transfer the wisdom of those leaders whom we interviewed to those in the field, and it provides a guide for building a career of impact, including action steps to do so. We encourage you to revisit these action steps, which appear at the end of each chapter, as you encounter the various types of issues inevitable in a career of impact. Make sure you complete the exercises. You will find that doing so helps you systematically break down the approach to leadership excellence at every stage of your career.

Great leadership potential is in all of us. We challenge healthcare leaders to adopt a personal action plan to further develop the seven building blocks for a career of impact. Apply them to enhance your legacy throughout your professional lives, and well into your encore performance.

American College of Healthcare Executives Code of Ethics*

PREAMBLE

The purpose of the *Code of Ethics* of the American College of Healthcare Executives is to serve as a standard of conduct for affiliates. It contains standards of ethical behavior for healthcare executives in their professional relationships. These relationships include colleagues, patients or others served; members of the healthcare executive's organization and other organizations; the community; and society as a whole.

The *Code of Ethics* also incorporates standards of ethical behavior governing individual behavior, particularly when that conduct directly relates to the role and identity of the healthcare executive.

The fundamental objectives of the healthcare management profession are to maintain or enhance the overall quality of life, dignity and well-being of every individual needing healthcare service and to create a more equitable, accessible, effective and efficient healthcare system.

Healthcare executives have an obligation to act in ways that will merit the trust, confidence, and respect of healthcare professionals

---

*As amended by the Board of Governors on November 14, 2011.

Source: Reprinted by permission of the American College of Healthcare Executives.

and the general public. Therefore, healthcare executives should lead lives that embody an exemplary system of values and ethics.

In fulfilling their commitments and obligations to patients or others served, healthcare executives function as moral advocates and models. Since every management decision affects the health and well-being of both individuals and communities, healthcare executives must carefully evaluate the possible outcomes of their decisions. In organizations that deliver healthcare services, they must work to safeguard and foster the rights, interests and prerogatives of patients or others served.

The role of moral advocate requires that healthcare executives take actions necessary to promote such rights, interests and prerogatives.

Being a model means that decisions and actions will reflect personal integrity and ethical leadership that others will seek to emulate.

Source: Reprinted by permission of the American College of Healthcare Executives.

I. THE HEALTHCARE EXECUTIVE'S RESPONSIBILITIES TO THE PROFESSION OF HEALTHCARE MANAGEMENT

The healthcare executive shall:

A. Uphold the *Code of Ethics* and mission of the American College of Healthcare Executives;

B. Conduct professional activities with honesty, integrity, respect, fairness and good faith in a manner that will reflect well upon the profession;

C. Comply with all laws and regulations pertaining to healthcare management in the jurisdictions in which the healthcare executive is located or conducts professional activities;

D. Maintain competence and proficiency in healthcare management by implementing a personal program of assessment and continuing professional education;

E. Avoid the improper exploitation of professional relationships for personal gain;

F. Disclose financial and other conflicts of interest;

G. Use this *Code* to further the interests of the profession and not for selfish reasons;

H. Respect professional confidences;

I. Enhance the dignity and image of the healthcare management profession through positive public information programs; and

J. Refrain from participating in any activity that demeans the credibility and dignity of the healthcare management profession.

Source: Reprinted by permission of the American College of Healthcare Executives.

II. THE HEALTHCARE EXECUTIVE'S RESPONSIBILITIES TO PATIENTS OR OTHERS SERVED

The healthcare executive shall, within the scope of his or her authority:

A. Work to ensure the existence of a process to evaluate the quality of care or service rendered;

B. Avoid practicing or facilitating discrimination and institute safeguards to prevent discriminatory organizational practices;

C. Work to ensure the existence of a process that will advise patients or others served of the rights, opportunities, responsibilities and risks regarding available healthcare services;

D. Work to ensure that there is a process in place to facilitate the resolution of conflicts that may arise when values of patients and their families differ from those of employees and physicians;

E. Demonstrate zero tolerance for any abuse of power that compromises patients or others served;

F. Work to provide a process that ensures the autonomy and self-determination of patients or others served;

G. Work to ensure the existence of procedures that will safeguard the confidentiality and privacy of patients or others served; and

H. Work to ensure the existence of an ongoing process and procedures to review, develop and consistently implement evidence-based clinical practices throughout the organization.

Source: Reprinted by permission of the American College of Healthcare Executives.

III. THE HEALTHCARE EXECUTIVE'S RESPONSIBILITIES TO THE ORGANIZATION

The healthcare executive shall, within the scope of his or her authority:

A. Provide healthcare services consistent with available resources, and when there are limited resources, work to ensure the existence of a resource allocation process that considers ethical ramifications;

B. Conduct both competitive and cooperative activities in ways that improve community healthcare services;

C. Lead the organization in the use and improvement of standards of management and sound business practices;

D. Respect the customs and practices of patients or others served, consistent with the organization's philosophy;

E. Be truthful in all forms of professional and organizational communication, and avoid disseminating information that is false, misleading or deceptive;

F. Report negative financial and other information promptly and accurately, and initiate appropriate action;

G. Prevent fraud and abuse and aggressive accounting practices that may result in disputable financial reports;

H. Create an organizational environment in which both clinical and management mistakes are minimized and, when they do occur, are disclosed and addressed effectively;

I. Implement an organizational code of ethics and monitor compliance; and

J. Provide ethics resources and mechanisms for staff to address ethical organizational and clinical issues.

Source: Reprinted by permission of the American College of Healthcare Executives.

IV. THE HEALTHCARE EXECUTIVE'S RESPONSIBILITIES TO EMPLOYEES

Healthcare executives have ethical and professional obligations to the employees they manage that encompass but are not limited to:

A. Creating a work environment that promotes ethical conduct;

B. Providing a work environment that encourages a free expression of ethical concerns and provides mechanisms for discussing and addressing such concerns;

C. Promoting a healthy work environment which includes freedom from harassment, sexual and other, and coercion of any kind, especially to perform illegal or unethical acts;

D. Promoting a culture of inclusivity that seeks to prevent discrimination on the basis of race, ethnicity, religion, gender, sexual orientation, age or disability;

E. Providing a work environment that promotes the proper use of employees' knowledge and skills; and

F. Providing a safe and healthy work environment.

Source: Reprinted by permission of the American College of Healthcare Executives.

V. THE HEALTHCARE EXECUTIVE'S RESPONSIBILITIES TO COMMUNITY AND SOCIETY

The healthcare executive shall:

A. Work to identify and meet the healthcare needs of the community;

B. Work to support access to healthcare services for all people;

C. Encourage and participate in public dialogue on healthcare policy issues, and advocate solutions that will improve health status and promote quality healthcare;

D. Apply short- and long-term assessments to management decisions affecting both community and society; and

E. Provide prospective patients and others with adequate and accurate information, enabling them to make enlightened decisions regarding services.

VI. THE HEALTHCARE EXECUTIVE'S RESPONSIBILITY TO REPORT VIOLATIONS OF THE *CODE*

An affiliate of ACHE who has reasonable grounds to believe that another affiliate has violated this *Code* has a duty to communicate such facts to the Ethics Committee.

Source: Reprinted by permission of the American College of Healthcare Executives.

ADDITIONAL RESOURCES

Available on **ache.org** or by calling ACHE at (312) 424-2800.

1. ACHE *Ethical Policy Statements*

   "Considerations for Healthcare Executive-Supplier Interactions"

   "Creating an Ethical Culture Within the Healthcare Organization"

   "Decisions Near the End of Life"

   "Ethical Decision Making for Healthcare Executives"

   "Ethical Issues Related to a Reduction in Force"

   "Ethical Issues Related to Staff Shortages"

   "Health Information Confidentiality"

   "Impaired Healthcare Executives"

   "Promise Making, Keeping and Rescinding"

2. ACHE Grievance Procedure

3. ACHE Ethics Committee Action

4. ACHE Ethics Committee Scope and Function

Source: Reprinted by permission of the American College of Healthcare Executives.

American College of Healthcare Executives
Policy Statement

Increasing and Sustaining Racial/Ethnic Diversity in Healthcare Management

July 1990
May 1995 (revised)
December 1998 (revised)
March 2002 (revised)
November 2005 (revised)
November 2010 (revised)

Statement of the Issue

One of the hallmarks of a democratic society is providing equal opportunity for all citizens regardless of race or ethnicity. In the healthcare sector, racially/ethnically diverse employees represent a growing percentage of all healthcare employees, but they hold only a modest percentage of top healthcare management positions. For example, according to the American Hospital Association, in 2010, 94 percent of all hospital CEOs were white[1] (non Hispanic or Latino) while 65 percent of the population is white[2] (non Hispanic or Latino), according to the most recent U.S. Census Bureau data.

Source: Reprinted by permission of the American College of Healthcare Executives.

This disparity persists despite two decades of success in attracting racially/ethnically diverse students to graduate study in health administration. For example, according to the Association of University Programs in Health Administration in 1990-1991, 14 percent of graduate students in healthcare management programs were racial/ethnic minorities. By the 2000-2001 academic year, the proportion rose to 30 percent and by 2009-2010, fully 42 percent of graduate students are minorities.[3]

In addition to these positive trends, a 2008 study[4] conducted jointly by the American College of Healthcare Executives (ACHE), the Asian Health Care Leaders Association, the Institute for Diversity in Health Management, the National Association of Health Services Executives, and the National Forum for Latino Healthcare Executives showed that among females, Latinos exceeded others in attaining senior-level positions. In regard to compensation levels, controlling for education and experience, black women earned similar incomes as white women. But Asian and Latino women earned about ten percent less than their white counterparts.

In the same study, the data for males shows that minority healthcare executives continue to earn less than their white counterparts. White males exceeded minorities in having attained senior-level positions in healthcare organizations and earned more than other racial/ethnic groups, when controlling for experience and education.

Our country's increasingly diverse communities result in a more diverse patient population. Studies suggest that diversity in healthcare management can enhance quality of care, quality of life in the workplace, community relations and the ability to affect community health status. Achieving diversity in management will involve a commitment at all professional levels (including early entrants, middle managers, and senior executives) within the organization through the awareness of diversity issues, hiring practices that attract diverse staff, development and mentoring in educational programs and organizations, and organization wide diversity training.

Source: Reprinted by permission of the American College of Healthcare Executives.

Policy Position

ACHE embraces diversity within the healthcare management field and recognizes that issue as both an ethical and business imperative. ACHE urges all healthcare executives, board members, educators and policymakers to actively strive to increase diversity within healthcare management ranks, especially in regard to race and ethnic background. ACHE actively strives to increase representation of racially/ethnically diverse individuals in healthcare management and works to create a supportive, collegial environment that encourages their membership and advancement within ACHE itself. ACHE, as a founding member, also is committed to collaborating with the Institute for Diversity in Health Management and other such groups on these issues.

All stakeholders should renew and strengthen their commitment to redressing any imbalance in representation of racially/ethnically diverse individuals in leadership to enhance our profession now and in the future.

ACHE encourages all healthcare executives to play a significant role in addressing this issue by actively pursuing the following:

Recruitment

- Promote healthcare careers to diverse populations via school programs and community organizations. Encourage students to shadow healthcare executives and explore careers in healthcare.
- Develop strong outreach mechanisms to attract promising racially/ethnically diverse candidates to healthcare management careers with special emphasis on increasing recruitment efforts at colleges and universities with predominately racially/ethnically diverse student enrollments.
- Offer internships, residencies and fellowships to racially/ethnically diverse students and provide mentoring to help prepare them for success in the job market.

Source: Reprinted by permission of the American College of Healthcare Executives.

- Advocate racial/ethnic diversity in the appointment of job search committee members and promote the provision of a diverse slate of candidates for senior management positions.
- Recruit racially/ethnically diverse individuals at every level, being transparent about hiring criteria, so as to increase current representation in management, but also to develop a pool of qualified candidates for the future.
- Recruit candidates external to the healthcare field to broaden the pool of racially/ethnically diverse candidates.
- Direct executive recruiters to identify and present racially/ethnically diverse candidates for management positions. Have them share criteria they use to recommend candidates for senior-level positions.

Promotion

- At every opportunity advocate the goal of achieving full representation of racially/ethnically diverse individuals at entry-, mid- and senior-levels in healthcare management.
- Institute policies that (1) prevent discrimination on the basis of race/ethnicity, (2) increase diversity in the recruitment and hiring of candidates, and (3) create an environment that encourages retention and promotion of qualified racially/ethnically diverse employees. Ensure that policies are well known and understood and measure and reward changes resulting from these policies.
- Consider utilizing pro-diversity initiatives to reduce social isolation through programs such as the following: appoint a manager responsible for diversity; appoint a diversity committee; adopt a diversity action plan; evaluate managers based on their diversity effectiveness; and promote social gatherings and mentoring programs.
- Publicize career advancement opportunities, such as continuing education, professional development organizations, networking

Source: Reprinted by permission of the American College of Healthcare Executives.

events and vacancies inside the organization, in a manner that appeals to everyone, especially racially/ethnically diverse individuals.

- Encourage retention and advancement of racially/ethnically diverse individuals. Identify potential candidates to support and create clear pathways for advancement from entry- to mid-level positions and from mid- to senior-level positions.
- Develop and disseminate specific criteria for advancement in management that would allow all individuals to have an equal opportunity for senior-level positions. Such criteria could be useful to racially/ethnically diverse individuals who wish to prepare themselves for senior-level positions.
- Conduct regular reviews of organizational compensation programs to ensure salaries are equitable and nondiscriminatory.

Support

- Work with organizations representing racially/ethnically diverse individuals within their communities to create sources for scholarships and fellowships.
- Advocate for governmental and private philanthropic programs that increase funding to underwrite advanced education, information dissemination and employment opportunities for racially/ethnically diverse individuals.
- Support organizations, such as the Institute for Diversity in Health Management, the Asian Health Care Leaders Association, the National Association of Health Services Executives and the National Forum for Latino Healthcare Executives that champion diverse executives through internships and other programming. Enable employed diverse executives to participate in the programs and be part of the volunteer leadership of such organizations.
- Support and assist the development of mentoring programs within healthcare organizations specifically focused on

Source: Reprinted by permission of the American College of Healthcare Executives.

developing long-term relationships between senior healthcare managers and racially/ethnically diverse candidates.

- Provide scholarship support for employed diverse executives to participate in leadership development programs.
- Urge racially/ethnically diverse healthcare executives who are not affiliates to join ACHE and become active at both the local (via chapters) and national levels. Extend invitations to hosted events such as executive breakfasts, chapter networking events and educational programs.

In addition, ACHE encourages racially/ethnically diverse healthcare executives to actively pursue the following:

- Earn an advanced degree in healthcare management or business.
- Seek internships, fellowships and administrative development opportunities that lead to permanent positions and form a foundation for building their careers.
- Seek positions in organizations that offer effective pro-diversity initiatives in order to build their careers.
- Choose positions that offer new experiences and expand their skillsets and management abilities.
- Interact with colleagues and actively pursue professional development by becoming involved in professional associations.
- Seek out mentors and serve as mentors to other professionals.

ACHE advocates a variety of approaches to improve the representation and equitable treatment of racial and ethnic diversity in healthcare management.

Approved by the Board of Governors of the American College of Healthcare Executives on November 8, 2010.

Source: Reprinted by permission of the American College of Healthcare Executives.

References

American Hospital Association, Division of Membership database. Accessed January 2010

U.S. Census Bureau, "Selected Social Characteristics in the United States." Accessed September 30, 2010

http://factfinder.census.gov

Association of University Programs in Health Administration 2008-09 Academic Program Survey

American College of Healthcare Executives, "2008 Racial/Ethnic Comparison of Career Attainments in Healthcare Management"

www.ache.org/PUBS/research/Report_Tables.pdf

Related Resources

American College of Healthcare Executives Diversity Resources: www.ache.org/policy/diversity_resources.cfm

Asian Health Care Leaders Association: www.asianhealthcareleaders.org

Institute for Diversity in Health Management: www.diversityconnection.org

National Association of Health Services Executives: www.nahse.org

National Forum for Latino Healthcare Executives: www.nflhe.org

Source: Reprinted by permission of the American College of Healthcare Executives.

American College of Healthcare Executives
Ethical Policy Statement

Creating an Ethical Culture
Within the Healthcare Organization

March 1992
August 1995 (revised)
November 2000 (revised)
November 2005 (revised)
November 2010 (revised)
November 2011 (revised)

Statement of the Issue

The number and significance of challenges facing healthcare organizations are unprecedented. Growing financial pressures, rising public and payor expectations, consolidations and mergers, patient safety and quality improvement issues, and healthcare reform have placed healthcare organizations under great stress—thus potentially intensifying ethics concerns and conflicts.

Healthcare organizations must be led and managed with integrity and consistent adherence to professional and ethical standards. The executive, in partnership with the board, and acting with other responsible parties such as ethics committees, must serve as a role

Source: Reprinted by permission of the American College of Healthcare Executives.

model and foster and support a culture that not only provides high-quality, cost-effective healthcare but promotes the ethical behavior and practices of individuals throughout the organization.

Recognizing the significance of ethics to the organization's mission and fulfillment of its responsibilities, healthcare executives must demonstrate the importance of ethics in their own actions and seek various ways to integrate ethical practices and reflection into the organization's culture. To create an ethical culture, healthcare executives should: 1) support the development and implementation of ethical standards of behavior including ethical clinical, management, research and quality-improvement practices; 2) ensure that effective and comprehensive ethics resources, including an ethics committee, exist and are available to develop, propagate and clarify such standards of behavior when there is ethical uncertainty; and 3) support and implement a systematic and organizationwide approach to ethics training and corporate compliance.

The ability of an organization to achieve its full potential will remain dependent upon the motivation, knowledge, skills, and ethical practices and values of each individual within the organization. Thus, the executive has an obligation to accomplish the organization's mission in a manner that respects the values of individuals and maximizes their contributions.

Policy Position

The American College of Healthcare Executives believes that all healthcare executives have a professional obligation to create an ethical working environment and culture. To this end, healthcare executives should lead these efforts by:

- Demonstrating and modeling the importance of and commitment to ethics through decisions, practices and behaviors;

Source: Reprinted by permission of the American College of Healthcare Executives.

- Promulgating an organizational code of ethics that includes ethical standards of behavior and guidelines;
- Reviewing the principles and ideals expressed in vision, mission and value statements, personnel policies, annual reports, orientation materials and other documents to ensure congruence;
- Supporting perspectives and behaviors that reflect that ethics is essential to achieving the organization's mission;
- Using communications throughout the year to help foster an understanding of the organization's commitment to ethics;
- Communicating expectations that behaviors and actions are based on the organization's code of ethics, values and ethical standards of practice. Such expectations should also be included in orientations and position descriptions where relevant;
- Ensuring that individuals throughout the organization are respected and expected to behave in an ethical manner;
- Fostering an environment where the free expression of ethical concerns is encouraged and supported without retribution;
- Ensuring that effective ethics resources, such as an ethics committee, are available for discussing and addressing clinical, organizational and research ethical concerns;
- Establishing a mechanism that safeguards individuals who wish to raise ethical concerns;
- Seeking to ensure that individuals are free from all harassment, coercion and discrimination;
- Providing an effective and timely process to facilitate dispute resolution;
- Using each individual's knowledge, skills and abilities appropriately; and
- Ensuring a safe work environment exists.

These responsibilities can best be implemented in an environment in which each individual within the organization is encouraged

Source: Reprinted by permission of the American College of Healthcare Executives.

and supported in adhering to the highest standards of ethics. This should be done with attention to the organization's code of ethics and appropriate professional codes, particularly those that stress the moral character and behavior of the executive and the organization itself.

Approved by the Board of Governors of the American College of Healthcare Executives on November 14, 2011.

Related Resources

American College of Healthcare Executives Ethics Toolkit

www.ache.org/ABT_ACHE/EthicsToolkit/ethicsTOC.cfm

Source: Reprinted by permission of the American College of Healthcare Executives.

American College of Healthcare Executives
Ethical Policy Statement

Ethical Decision Making for Healthcare Executives

August 1993
February 1997 (revised)
November 2002 (revised)
November 2007 (revised)
November 2011 (revised)

Statement of the Issue

Ethical decision making is required when the healthcare executive must address a conflict or uncertainty regarding competing values, such as personal, organizational, professional and societal values. Those involved in this decision-making process must consider ethical principles including justice, autonomy, beneficence and nonmaleficence as well as professional and organizational ethical standards and codes. Many factors have contributed to the growing concern in healthcare organizations over ethical issues, including issues of access and affordability, pressure to reduce costs, mergers and acquisitions, financial and other resource constraints, and advances in medical technology that complicate decision making

Source: Reprinted by permission of the American College of Healthcare Executives.

near the end of life. Healthcare executives have a responsibility to address the growing number of complex ethical dilemmas they are facing, but they cannot and should not make such decisions alone or without a sound decision-making framework.

Healthcare organizations should have mechanisms that may include ethics committees, ethics consultation services, and written policies, procedures and guidelines to assist them with the ethics decision-making process. With these organizational mechanisms and guidelines in place, conflicting interests involving patients, families, caregivers, the organization, payors and the community can be thoughtfully and appropriately reviewed.

Policy Position

It is incumbent upon healthcare executives to lead in a manner that sets an ethical tone for their organizations. The American College of Healthcare Executives (ACHE) believes that education in ethics is an important step in a healthcare executive's lifelong commitment to high ethical conduct, both personally and professionally. Further, ACHE supports the development of organizational mechanisms that enable healthcare executives to appropriately and expeditiously address ethical conflicts. Whereas physicians, nurses and other caregivers may primarily address ethical issues on a case-by-case basis, healthcare executives also have a responsibility to address those issues at broader organizational, community and societal levels. ACHE encourages its affiliates, as leaders in their organizations, to take an active role in the development and demonstration of ethical decision making.

To this end, healthcare executives should:

- Create a culture that fosters ethical clinical and administrative practices and ethical decision making.

Source: Reprinted by permission of the American College of Healthcare Executives.

- Communicate the organization's commitment to ethical decision making through its mission or value statements and its organizational code of ethics.
- Demonstrate through their professional behavior the importance of ethics to the organization.
- Offer educational programs to boards, staff, physicians and others on their organization's ethical standards of practice and on the more global issues of ethical decision making in today's healthcare environment. Further, healthcare executives should promote learning opportunities, such as those provided through professional societies or academic organizations, that will facilitate open discussion of ethical issues.
- Develop and use organizational mechanisms that reflect their organizations' mission and values and are flexible enough to deal with the spectrum of ethical concerns—clinical, organizational, business and management.
- Ensure that organizational mechanisms to address ethics issues are readily available and include individuals who are competent to address ethical concerns and reflect diverse perspectives. An organization's ethics committee, for example, might include representatives from groups such as physicians, nurses, managers, board members, social workers, attorneys, patients and/or the community and clergy. All these groups are likely to bring unique and valuable perspectives to bear on discussions of ethical issues.
- Evaluate and continually refine organizational processes for addressing ethical issues.
- Promote decision making that results in the appropriate use of power while balancing individual, organizational and societal issues.

Approved by the Board of Governors of the American College of Healthcare Executives on November 14, 2011.

Source: Reprinted by permission of the American College of Healthcare Executives.

American College of Healthcare Executives
Ethical Policy Statement

Ethical Issues Related to a Reduction in Force

August 1995
November 2000 (revised)
November 2005 (revised)

Statement of the Issue

As the result of managed care, such as variable admissions, shorter lengths of stay, higher productivity, new technology, and other factors, the capacity of some healthcare organizations could significantly exceed demand. As a result, these organizations may be required to reduce their work force. Additionally, mergers and consolidations can result in further reductions and reassignments of staff. Financial pressures will continue to fuel this trend. However, patient care needs should not be compromised when determining staffing requirements.

Careful planning, diligent cost controls, effective resource management, and proper consultation can lessen the hardship and stress of a reduction in force. Formal policies and procedures should be developed well in advance of the need to implement them.

Source: Reprinted by permission of the American College of Healthcare Executives.

The decision to reduce staff necessitates consideration of the short-term and long-term impact on all employees—those leaving and those remaining. Decision makers should consider the potential ethical conflict between formally stated organizational values and staff reduction actions.

Policy Position

The American College of Healthcare Executives recommends that specific steps be considered by healthcare executives when initiating a reduction in force process to support consistency between stated organizational values and those demonstrated before, during and after the process. Among these steps are the following:

- Recognize that cost reduction efforts must be appropriate—if they are too aggressive, the consequences for patients, staff and the organization can be as harmful as doing too little or proceeding too late;
- Consult with labor counsel;
- Provide timely, accurate, clear and consistent information—including the reasoning behind the decision—to stakeholders when staff reductions become necessary;
- Review the principles and ideals expressed in vision, mission and value statements, personnel policies, annual reports, employee orientation materials, and other documents to test congruence and conformance with reduction in force decisions;
- Support, if possible, through retraining and redeployment, employees whose positions have been eliminated. Also, consider outplacement assistance and appropriate severance policies, if possible; and
- Address the needs of remaining staff by demonstrating sensitivity to their potential feelings of loss, anger and survivor

Source: Reprinted by permission of the American College of Healthcare Executives.

guilt. Also address their anxiety about the possibility of further reductions, uncertainty regarding changes in workload, work redesign, and similar concerns.

Healthcare organizations encounter the same set of challenging issues associated with reductions in force as do other employers. Reduction in force decisions should reflect an institution's ethics and value statements.

Approved by the Board of Governors of the American College of Healthcare Executives on November 7, 2005.

Source: Reprinted by permission of the American College of Healthcare Executives.

American College of Healthcare Executives
Ethical Policy Statement

Impaired Healthcare Executives

February 1991
March 1995 (revised)
November 2000 (revised)
November 2005 (revised)
November 2006 (revised)

Statement of the Issue

The American College of Healthcare Executives recognizes that impairment, defined broadly to include alcoholism, substance abuse, chemical dependency, mental/emotional instability or cognitive impairment, is a significant problem that crosses all societal boundaries.

Impairment occurs when the healthcare executive is unable to perform professional duties as expected. Impaired healthcare executives affect not only themselves and their families, but they also have a significant impact on their profession; their professional society; their organizations, colleagues, patients, clients and others served; their communities; and society as a whole. Impairment typically leads to misconduct in the form of incompetence and unsafe or unprofessional behavior, which also can lead to substantial costs associated with loss of productivity and errors in judgment.

Source: Reprinted by permission of the American College of Healthcare Executives.

The impaired healthcare executive can damage the public image of his or her organization of employment. Public confidence in the organization diminishes if it appears that the organization is not being managed with consistently high standards of professional and ethical practice. This lack of public confidence may cause the community to deem the organization unworthy of its support.

Society expects healthcare executives to practice the standards of good health that they advocate for the public. Impaired healthcare executives diminish the credibility of the profession and its ability to manage society's healthcare when they are not appropriately managing their own personal health.

Policy Position

The preamble of the American College of Healthcare Executives *Code of Ethics* states, "Healthcare executives have an obligation to act in ways that will merit the trust, confidence and respect of healthcare professionals and the general public. To do this, healthcare executives must lead lives that embody an exemplary system of values and ethics."

The American College of Healthcare Executives believes that all healthcare executives have an ethical and a professional obligation to:

- Maintain a personal health that is free from impairment.
- Refrain from all professional activities if impaired.
- Expeditiously seek treatment if impairment occurs.
- Urge impaired colleagues to expeditiously seek treatment and to refrain from all professional activities while impaired.
- Assist recovered colleagues when they resume their professional activities.

Source: Reprinted by permission of the American College of Healthcare Executives.

- Intervene and report the impairment to the appropriate person(s) should the colleague refuse to seek professional assistance and should the state of impairment persist.
- Support peers who identify healthcare executives in need of help.
- Recognize that individuals who have successfully received treatment for impairment and are no longer deemed impaired should be considered for employment opportunities for which they are qualified.
- Recommend or provide, within one's employing organization, confidential avenues for reporting impairment and either access or referral to treatment or assistance programs.
- Urge the community to provide information and resources for assistance and treatment of alcoholism, substance abuse, mental/emotional instability and cognitive impairment as needed and as appropriate.
- Raise the awareness of key stakeholders (such as employees, governing board members, etc.) on impairment issues and the resources available for assistance.

Approved by the Board of Governors of the American College of Healthcare Executives on November 6, 2006.

Source: Reprinted by permission of the American College of Healthcare Executives.

American College of Healthcare Executives
Policy Statement

Responsibility for Mentoring

November 1994
November 1999 (revised)
November 2004 (revised)
November 2009 (revised)

Statement of the Issue

The future of healthcare management rests in large measure with those entering the field as well as with mid-careerists who aspire to new and greater management opportunities. While on-the-job experience and continuing education are critical elements for preparing tomorrow's leaders, the value of mentoring these individuals cannot be overstated. Growing through mentoring relationships is an important factor in a protégé's lifelong learning process. In turn, by sharing their wisdom, insights and experiences, mentors can give back to the profession while deriving the personal satisfaction that comes from helping others realize their potential. For the organization, mentorships can lead to more satisfied employees and the generation of new ideas and programs.

Source: Reprinted by permission of the American College of Healthcare Executives.

Policy Position

The American College of Healthcare Executives (ACHE) believes that healthcare executives have a professional obligation to mentor both those entering the field and mid-careerists preparing to lead the healthcare systems of tomorrow.

Experienced healthcare executives can provide guidance to others in many ways, including:

Assisting Students and Those Entering the Field

- Offer assistance by recruiting, interviewing and working with qualified students interested in pursuing healthcare management careers, including addressing their questions relative to pursuing appropriate ongoing education or a graduate degree.
- Volunteer to serve as a guest lecturer, and use this opportunity to provide students with career planning guidance and insights gleaned from past experience.
- Offer externships, internships, residencies and postgraduate fellowships.
- Provide meaningful first-job opportunities to promising graduates and counsel them along the way.

Engaging in and Supporting Mentoring Relationships

- Promote mentoring opportunities and an organizational culture that promotes mentoring.
- Help protégés develop clear expectations about their role so they will actively contribute to the mentoring relationship.
- Encourage development of mentoring opportunities in culturally diverse, cross-generational and group settings as well as among individuals of different genders, races and ethnicities.

Source: Reprinted by permission of the American College of Healthcare Executives.

- Encourage other experienced executives from across the spectrum of healthcare organizations to engage in mentoring relationships.
- Keep abreast of changes in mentoring philosophy and techniques so as to ensure continued effectiveness as a mentor in an environment characterized by profound and rapid change.
- Seek out opportunities to contribute to local independent chapters of ACHE.

By providing guidance and engaging in mentoring relationships, healthcare leaders can benefit their organizations, contribute to the future of the profession and gain the personal gratification of helping less experienced individuals grow professionally.

Approved by the Board of Governors of the American College of Healthcare Executives on November 16, 2009.

Source: Reprinted by permission of the American College of Healthcare Executives.

American College of Healthcare Executives
Policy Statement

Preventing and Addressing Workplace Abuse: Inappropriate and Disruptive Behavior

November 1996
November 1999 (revised)
November 2002 (revised)
November 2005 (reaffirmed)
November 2010 (revised)

Statement of the Issue

Healthcare executives have a professional responsibility to create and maintain an organizational culture that promotes quality patient care and a healthy work environment that protects staff from inappropriate and disruptive behavior. Such behavior, including aggression, harassment and intimidation, can adversely affect the ability of the healthcare team to work together and can negatively impact the quality of patient care. Countering the adverse effects of inappropriate and disruptive behavior requires that healthcare executives

Source: Reprinted by permission of the American College of Healthcare Executives.

establish an organizational code of conduct defining such behaviors, provide staff with relevant education, and implement enforceable policies and processes to identify and prevent such behaviors.

An organizational culture that clearly conveys zero tolerance for inappropriate and disruptive behaviors while providing the necessary resources and mechanisms to safeguard against such behaviors can improve teamwork, foster a sense of mutual respect, and improve communication. Not only can quality of care and patient safety be enhanced, but there is a concomitant reduction in the legal, physical and emotional repercussions of inappropriate and disruptive behavior such as loss of productivity, absenteeism, turnover, low morale, lack of trust, communication breakdowns, and long-term career and psychological damage.

Policy Position

The American College of Healthcare Executives believes that all healthcare executives have a professional and ethical responsibility to promote a healthy workplace that is free of aggression, harassment and intimidation. Healthcare executives should demonstrate zero tolerance for inappropriate and disruptive behavior, including harassment on the basis of gender, sexual orientation, age, race, ethnicity, religion, national origin, disability, or any other personal characteristic. On behalf of their employing organizations, healthcare executives must further realize that they are responsible for implementing policy and monitoring compliance among their managers. To this end, healthcare executives should model desired behaviors and promote multifaceted programs in their organizations to prevent inappropriate and disruptive behaviors. Sample program components include, but are not limited to, the following:

Clearly articulated code of conduct and policy against inappropriate and disruptive behavior. The organization should have

Source: Reprinted by permission of the American College of Healthcare Executives.

a code of conduct that defines acceptable, disruptive and inappropriate behavior. The related policy also should define specific
terms such as "harassment" (preferably as defined by the Equal
Employment Opportunity Commission–EEOC) and "aggression,"
and reference intimidation (both verbal and non-verbal), violence
(both physical and verbal) and passive aggressive behaviors. In addition, the policy should explicitly state that these behaviors are not
tolerated in the organization. The policy might include examples of
prohibited conduct, delineate methods for making and investigating
complaints, state that retaliation is prohibited and no reprisals will
be taken against any employee filing a complaint under this policy,
and provide that appropriate corrective action will be taken. The
code of conduct and policy should be revised on a periodic basis
and incorporated into the employee handbook as well as discussed
in new employee orientation.

**Employee training on inappropriate and disruptive behavior
and its prevention.** Human resources staff or other individuals who
have a technical and legal understanding of the issues, in addition
to demonstrated ability to stimulate discussion about this sensitive
topic should conduct training. Training should be conducted on
an ongoing and regular basis with the goals of: raising awareness of
harassment, intimidation and aggression; clarifying misconceptions
about what constitutes these behaviors; explaining the manager's
role and responsibility in providing a safe and supportive work
environment; and finally, sharing the specifics of the organization's
policy prohibiting inappropriate and disruptive behavior.

**Procedure for reporting allegations of inappropriate and dis-
ruptive behavior.** The procedure should provide as much confidentiality as possible for both the complaining employee and the
person accused of these behaviors. The procedure should take into
account the need of the individual accused to be presented with
the specific charges so as to be able to form a defense. Employees

Source: Reprinted by permission of the American College of Healthcare Executives.

should be protected from retaliation for filing a complaint or appearing as a witness in an investigation. Further, if the procedure requires employees to make initial complaints to their supervisors, an alternate person should be designated to handle complaints when lodged against the supervisor. Supervisors should be required to report all complaints and be made aware of liability for failing to do so.

Procedure for expeditiously investigating complaints of inappropriate and disruptive behavior. According to EEOC guidelines, once an employee complains, employers should promptly investigate and take "immediate and appropriate corrective action" based upon the results of their investigation. The organization should, therefore, have a process in place for investigating complaints quickly, discreetly and completely. An objective party should conduct an investigation, and the results of the investigation should be reported to both the complaining employee and the person accused. Other staff should be informed on a "need to know" basis.

Standards for corrective action. Standards for corrective action are an essential part of any plan to prevent inappropriate and disruptive behavior. Disciplinary action should be proportionate to the severity of any behavior found. The organization's policy, as it relates to corrective action, should avoid providing specific punishments for specific actions and instead be broad enough to give the freedom to exercise appropriate action. For example, the policy might state that such behaviors may result in discipline, up to and including discharge.

In addition to the program components mentioned above, legal counsel should review policies and procedures related to inappropriate and disruptive behavior because of the potential exposure to liability.

Source: Reprinted by permission of the American College of Healthcare Executives.

Workplace safety and quality of patient care is dependent on teamwork, communication and a collaborative work environment. To assure quality and to promote a culture of safety, healthcare executives must address the continuum of inappropriate behaviors that threaten overall performance and patient outcomes.

Approved by the Board of Governors of the American College of Healthcare Executives on November 8, 2010.

References

American Medical Association's Opinion E-9.045

The Joint Commission Standard L.D. 03.01.01 www.jointcommission.org/NewsRoom/PressKits/Behaviors+that+Undermine+a+Culture+of+Safety/

The Joint Commission, Sentinel Event Alert, Issue 40 www.jointcommission.org/SentinelEvents/

Related Resources

American College of Physician Executives, "Special Report: 2009 Doctor-Nurse Behavior Survey," The Physician Executive, November/December 2009, Vol. 35, Issue 6 www.ache.org/policy/doctornursebehavior.pdf

Source: Reprinted by permission of the American College of Healthcare Executives.

Ethics Self-Assessment

Purpose of the Ethics Self-Assessment

Members of the American College of Healthcare Executives agree, as a condition of membership, to abide by ACHE's *Code of Ethics.* The *Code* provides an overall standard of conduct and includes specific standards of ethical behavior to guide healthcare executives in their professional relationships.

Based on the *Code of Ethics,* the Ethics Self-Assessment is intended for your personal use to assist you in thinking about your ethics-related leadership and actions. *It should not be returned to ACHE nor should it be used as a tool for evaluating the ethical behavior of others.*

The Ethics Self-Assessment can help you identify those areas in which you are on strong ethical ground; areas that you may wish to examine the basis for your responses; and opportunities for further reflection. The Ethics Self-Assessment does not have a scoring mechanism, as we do not believe that ethical behavior can or should be quantified.

How to Use This Self-Assessment

We hope you find this self-assessment thought provoking and useful as a part of your reflection on applying the ACHE *Code of Ethics* to

Source: Reprinted by permission of the American College of Healthcare Executives.

your everyday activities. You are to be commended for taking time out of your busy schedule to complete it.

Once you have finished the self-assessment, it is suggested that you review your responses, noting which questions you answered "usually," "occasionally" and "almost never." You may find that in some cases an answer of "usually" is satisfactory, but in other cases such as when answering a question about protecting staff's well-being, an answer of "usually" may raise an ethical red flag.

We are confident that you will uncover few red flags where your responses are not compatible with the ACHE *Code of Ethics.* For those you may discover, you should use this as an opportunity to enhance your ethical practice and leadership by developing a specific action plan. For example, you may have noted in the self-assessment that you have not used your organization's ethics mechanism to assist you in addressing challenging ethical conflicts. As a result of this insight you might meet with the chair of the ethics committee to better understand the committee's functions, including case consultation activities, and how you might access this resource when future ethical conflicts arise.

We also want you to consider ACHE as a resource when you and your management team are confronted with difficult ethical dilemmas. In the About ACHE area of **ache.org,** you can access an Ethics Toolkit, a group of practical resources that will help you understand how to integrate ethics into your organization. In addition, you can refer to our regular "Healthcare Management Ethics" column in *Healthcare Executive* magazine, and you may want to consider attending our annual ethics seminar.

Source: Reprinted by permission of the American College of Healthcare Executives.

Please check one answer for each of the following questions.

	Almost Never	Occasionally	Usually	Always	Not Applicable
I. LEADERSHIP					
I take courageous, consistent and appropriate management actions to overcome barriers to achieving my organization's mission.	☐	☐	☐	☐	☐
I place community/patient benefit over my personal gain.	☐	☐	☐	☐	☐
I strive to be a role model for ethical behavior.	☐	☐	☐	☐	☐
I work to ensure that decisions about access to care are based primarily on medical necessity, not only on the ability to pay.	☐	☐	☐	☐	☐
My statements and actions are consistent with professional ethical standards, including the ACHE *Code of Ethics*.	☐	☐	☐	☐	☐
My statements and actions are honest even when circumstances would allow me to confuse the issues.	☐	☐	☐	☐	☐
I advocate ethical decision making by the board, management team and medical staff.	☐	☐	☐	☐	☐
I use an ethical approach to conflict resolution.	☐	☐	☐	☐	☐
I initiate and encourage discussion of the ethical aspects of management/financial issues.	☐	☐	☐	☐	☐

Source: Reprinted by permission of the American College of Healthcare Executives.

	Almost Never	Occasionally	Usually	Always	Not Applicable
I initiate and promote discussion of controversial issues affecting community/patient health (e.g., domestic and community violence and decisions near the end of life).	❑	❑	❑	❑	❑
I promptly and candidly explain to internal and external stakeholders negative economic trends and encourage appropriate action.	❑	❑	❑	❑	❑
I use my authority solely to fulfill my responsibilities and not for self-interest or to further the interests of family, friends or associates.	❑	❑	❑	❑	❑
When an ethical conflict confronts my organization or me, I am successful in finding an effective resolution process and ensure it is followed.	❑	❑	❑	❑	❑
I demonstrate respect for my colleagues, superiors and staff.	❑	❑	❑	❑	❑
I demonstrate my organization's vision, mission and value statements in my actions.	❑	❑	❑	❑	❑
I make timely decisions rather than delaying them to avoid difficult or politically risky choices.	❑	❑	❑	❑	❑
I seek the advice of the ethics committee when making ethically challenging decisions.	❑	❑	❑	❑	❑
My personal expense reports are accurate and are only billed to a single organization.	❑	❑	❑	❑	❑

Source: Reprinted by permission of the American College of Healthcare Executives.

	Almost Never	Occasionally	Usually	Always	Not Applicable
I openly support establishing and monitoring internal mechanisms (e.g., an ethics committee or program) to support ethical decision making.	❏	❏	❏	❏	❏
I thoughtfully consider decisions when making a promise on behalf of the organization to a person or a group of people.	❏	❏	❏	❏	❏

II. RELATIONSHIPS
Community

	Almost Never	Occasionally	Usually	Always	Not Applicable
I promote community health status improvement as a guiding goal of my organization and as a cornerstone of my efforts on behalf of my organization.	❏	❏	❏	❏	❏
I personally devote time to developing solutions to community health problems.	❏	❏	❏	❏	❏
I participate in and encourage my management team to devote personal time to community service.	❏	❏	❏	❏	❏

Patients and Their Families

	Almost Never	Occasionally	Usually	Always	Not Applicable
I use a patient- and family-centered approach to patient care.	❏	❏	❏	❏	❏
I am a patient advocate on both clinical and financial matters.	❏	❏	❏	❏	❏
I ensure equitable treatment of patients regardless of their socioeconomic status, ethnicity or payor category.	❏	❏	❏	❏	❏

Source: Reprinted by permission of the American College of Healthcare Executives.

	Almost Never	Occasionally	Usually	Always	Not Applicable
I respect the practices and customs of a diverse patient population while maintaining the organization's mission.	❑	❑	❑	❑	❑
I demonstrate through organizational policies and personal actions that overtreatment and undertreatment of patients are unacceptable.	❑	❑	❑	❑	❑
I protect patients' rights to autonomy through access to full, accurate information about their illnesses, treatment options and related costs and benefits.	❑	❑	❑	❑	❑
I promote a patient's right to privacy, including medical record confidentiality, and do not tolerate breaches of this confidentiality.	❑	❑	❑	❑	❑

Board

	Almost Never	Occasionally	Usually	Always	Not Applicable
I have a routine system in place for board members to make full disclosure and reveal potential conflicts of interest.	❑	❑	❑	❑	❑
I ensure that reports to the board, my own or others', appropriately convey risks of decisions or proposed projects.	❑	❑	❑	❑	❑
I work to keep the board focused on ethical issues of importance to the organization, community and other stakeholders.	❑	❑	❑	❑	❑

Source: Reprinted by permission of the American College of Healthcare Executives.

	Almost Never	Occasionally	Usually	Always	Not Applicable
I keep the board appropriately informed of patient safety and quality indicators.	❏	❏	❏	❏	❏
I promote board discussion of resource allocation issues, particularly those where organizational and community interests may appear to be incompatible.	❏	❏	❏	❏	❏
I keep the board appropriately informed about issues of alleged financial malfeasance, clinical malpractice and potential litigious situations involving employees.	❏	❏	❏	❏	❏

Colleagues and Staff

	Almost Never	Occasionally	Usually	Always	Not Applicable
I foster discussions about ethical concerns when they arise.	❏	❏	❏	❏	❏
I maintain confidences entrusted to me.	❏	❏	❏	❏	❏
I demonstrate through personal actions and organizational policies zero tolerance for any form of staff harassment.	❏	❏	❏	❏	❏
I encourage discussions about and advocate for the implementation of the organization's code of ethics and value statements.	❏	❏	❏	❏	❏
I fulfill the promises I make.	❏	❏	❏	❏	❏
I am respectful of views different from mine.	❏	❏	❏	❏	❏

Source: Reprinted by permission of the American College of Healthcare Executives.

	Almost Never	Occasionally	Usually	Always	Not Applicable
I am respectful of individuals who differ from me in ethnicity, gender, education or job position.	❑	❑	❑	❑	❑
I convey negative news promptly and openly, not allowing employees or others to be misled.	❑	❑	❑	❑	❑
I expect and hold staff accountable for adherence to our organization's ethical standards (e.g., performance reviews).	❑	❑	❑	❑	❑
I demonstrate that incompetent supervision is not tolerated and make timely decisions regarding marginally performing managers.	❑	❑	❑	❑	❑
I ensure adherence to ethics-related policies and practices affecting patients and staff.	❑	❑	❑	❑	❑
I am sensitive to employees who have ethical concerns and facilitate resolution of these concerns.	❑	❑	❑	❑	❑
I encourage the use of organizational mechanisms (e.g., an ethics committee or program) and other ethics resources to address ethical issues.	❑	❑	❑	❑	❑
I act quickly and decisively when employees are not treated fairly in their relationships with other employees.	❑	❑	❑	❑	❑

Source: Reprinted by permission of the American College of Healthcare Executives.

	Almost Never	Occasionally	Usually	Always	Not Applicable
I assign staff only to official duties and do not ask them to assist me with work on behalf of my family, friends or associates.	☐	☐	☐	☐	☐
I hold all staff and clinical/business partners accountable for compliance with professional standards, including ethical behavior.	☐	☐	☐	☐	☐

Clinicians

	Almost Never	Occasionally	Usually	Always	Not Applicable
When problems arise with clinical care, I ensure that the problems receive prompt attention and resolution by the responsible parties.	☐	☐	☐	☐	☐
I insist that my organization's clinical practice guidelines are consistent with our vision, mission, value statements and ethical standards of practice.	☐	☐	☐	☐	☐
When practice variations in care suggest quality of care is at stake, I encourage timely actions that serve patients' interests.	☐	☐	☐	☐	☐
I insist that participating clinicians and staff live up to the terms of managed care contracts.	☐	☐	☐	☐	☐
I encourage clinicians to access ethics resources when ethical conflicts occur.	☐	☐	☐	☐	☐

Source: Reprinted by permission of the American College of Healthcare Executives.

	Almost Never	Occasionally	Usually	Always	Not Applicable
I encourage resource allocation that is equitable, is based on clinical needs and appropriately balances patient needs and organizational/ clinical resources.	❑	❑	❑	❑	❑
I expeditiously and forthrightly deal with impaired clinicians and take necessary action when I believe a clinician is not competent to perform his/her clinical duties.	❑	❑	❑	❑	❑
I expect and hold clinicians accountable for adhering to their professional and the organization's ethical practices.	❑	❑	❑	❑	❑

Buyers, Payors and Suppliers

	Almost Never	Occasionally	Usually	Always	Not Applicable
I negotiate and expect my management team to negotiate in good faith.	❑	❑	❑	❑	❑
I am mindful of the importance of avoiding even the appearance of wrongdoing, conflict of interest, or interference with free competition.	❑	❑	❑	❑	❑
I personally disclose and expect board members, staff members and clinicians to disclose any possible conflicts of interest before pursuing or entering into relationships with potential business partners.	❑	❑	❑	❑	❑

Source: Reprinted by permission of the American College of Healthcare Executives.

	Almost Never	Occasionally	Usually	Always	Not Applicable
I promote familiarity and compliance with organizational policies governing relationships with buyers, payors and suppliers.	☐	☐	☐	☐	☐
I set an example for others in my organization by not accepting personal gifts from suppliers.	☐	☐	☐	☐	☐

Source: Reprinted by permission of the American College of Healthcare Executives.

References

Armada, A. A., and M. F. Hubbard. 2010. "Diversity in Healthcare: Time to Get REAL." *Frontiers of Health Services Management* 26 (3): 3–17.

Atchison, T. 2004. *Followership: A Practical Guide to Aligning Leaders and Followers*. Chicago: Health Administration Press.

Bach, D. 2005. *Start Late, Finish Rich*. New York: Random House.

Barsh, J., M. M. Capozzi, and J. Davidson. 2008. "Leadership and Innovation." *McKinsey Quarterly*. Published in January. www.mckinseyquarterly.com/ Leadership_and_innovation_2009.

Bauer-Maglin, N., and A. Radosh. 2003. *Women Confronting Retirement: A Nontraditional Guide*. Piscataway, NJ: Rutgers University Press.

Bluestone, B., and M. Melnik. 2010. "After the Recovery: Help Needed." *Civic Ventures*. Published March 22. www.encore.org/learn/emerging-encore-careers.

Brooks, D. 2007. "Time to Do Everything Except Think." *Newsweek*. Updated December 17 from original, published April 29, 2001. www.newsweek.com/ id/79934/output/print.

Carstensen, L. L. 2001. "On the Brink of a Brand-New Old Age." *New York Times*. Published January 2. http://www.nytimes.com/2001/01/02/opinion/ on-the-brink-of-a-brand-new-old-age.html?pagewanted=all&src=pm.

Center for Innovation. 2012. "Design Thinking." *Mayo Foundation for Education and Research*. Accessed May 10. www.mayo.edu/center-for-innovation/ what-we-do/design-thinking.

Charan, R. 2008a. *Leaders at All Levels*. San Francisco: Wiley & Sons.

———. 2008b. *The Leadership Pipeline: How to Build the Leadership-Powered Company*. San Francisco: Wiley & Sons.

Collins, J. 2001. *Good to Great: Why Some Companies Make the Leap . . . and Others Don't*. New York: Harper Business.

———. 1997. "The Most Creative Product Ever." Published in May. www.jimcollins.com/article_topics/articles/the-most-creative.html.

Connecticut Mentoring Partnership and Business and Legal Reports Inc. 1999. *Best Practices in Human Resources* 653 (September 30).

Cook, B. 2010. "Hospitals' New Specialist: Social Media Manager." *American Medical News* (November): 8.

Cordova, R. D., C. L. Beaudin, and K. E. Iwanabe. 2010. "Addressing Diversity and Moving Toward Equity in Hospital Care." *Frontiers of Health Services Management* 26 (3): 19–34.

Crom, S. 2012. "Dispelling Myths About Leadership Change." *The TRIZJournal.* Accessed April 11. www.triz-journal.com/content/c081006a.asp.

Cullinane, J., and C. Fitzgerald. 2007. *The New Retirement.* Emmaus, PA: Rodale.

Dunn, R. T. 2010. *Dunn & Haimann's Healthcare Management,* 9th ed. Chicago: Health Administration Press.

Freedman, M. 2010. "Choosing to Work During Retirement and the Impact on Social Security." Testimony to US Senate Committee on Finance, July 15. www.encore.org/find/resources/testimony-marc-freedman.

———. 2007. *Encore: Finding Work That Matters in the Second Half of Life.* New York: Public Affairs.

Freund, L. 2010. "Creating a Culture of Accountability." *Healthcare Executive* 31 (1): 30–36.

Galford, R. M., and R. F. Maruca. 2006. *Your Leadership Legacy.* Boston: Harvard Business School Press.

Garman, A. N., T. J. Johnson, and T. C. Royer. 2011. *The Future of Healthcare: Global Trends Worth Watching.* Chicago: Health Administration Press.

George, B. 2003. *Authentic Leadership: Rediscovering the Secrets to Creating Lasting Value.* San Francisco: Jossey-Bass.

Goldsmith, M. 2009. *Succession: Are You Ready?* Boston: Harvard Business School Press.

Goleman, D. 1992. *Working with Emotional Intelligence.* New York: Bantam.

Gostick, A., and C. Elton. 2007. *The Carrot Principle.* New York: Free Press.

Govindarajan, V., and S. Peters. 2011. "Embedding Innovation in Leadership." *Businessweek.* Published February 1. www.businessweek.com/managing/content/jan2011/ca20110131_365732.htm.

Grant, S. 2010. "Diversity in Healthcare: Driven by Leadership." *Frontiers of Health Services Management* 26 (3): 41–44.

Health Research & Educational Trust (HRET) and Institute for Diversity in Healthcare Management (IFD). 2011. "Building a Culturally Competent Organization: The Quest for Equity in Health Care." Chicago: HRET.

Hesselbein, F., and A. Shrader. 2008. *Leader to Leader: Enduring Insights on Leadership.* San Francisco: Jossey-Bass.

Hofmann, P. B. 2011. "Culture Clashes and Moral Judgments." *Healthcare Executive* 26 (1): 52–55.

———. 2010. "Addressing Racial and Ethnic Disparities in Healthcare." *Healthcare Executive* 25 (5): 46–50.

Horth, D., and D. Buchner. 2009. "Innovation Leadership: How to Use Innovation to Lead Effectively, Work Collaboratively and Drive Results." *Center for Creative Leadership and Continuum.* Accessed May 10, 2012. www.ccl.org/leadership/pdf/research/InnovationLeadership.pdf.

Institute of Medicine (IOM). 2004. *In the Nation's Compelling Interest: Ensuring Diversity in the Health Care Workforce.* Washington, DC: National Academies Press.

————. 2000. *Toward a New Definition of Diversity.* Washington, DC: National Academies Press.

Integrated Health Strategies (IHS). n.d. "Leadership Continuity Services." *IHS.* Accessed May 10, 2012. www.ihstrategies.com/articles/274.pdf.

Kouzes, J. M., and B. Z. Posner. 2006. *A Leader's Legacy.* San Francisco: Jossey-Bass.

————. 1993. *Credibility: How Leaders Gain and Lose It, Why People Demand It.* San Francisco: Jossey-Bass.

LaFasto, F., and C. Larson. 2001. *When Teams Work Best: 6,000 Team Members and Leaders Tell What It Takes to Succeed.* Thousand Oaks, CA: Sage.

Lancaster, L., and D. Stillman. 2011. "What a Difference a Generation Makes." Presentation at BridgeWorks Spring Conference, Chicago, March 7.

Lipman, J. 2011. "Are Ethics for Suckers?" *Newsweek*, April 10, p. 8.

Lloyd, M. 2009. *Super-Charged Retirement: Ditch the Rocking Chair, Trash the Remote, and Do What You Love.* Austin, TX: Greenleaf Book Group.

Maruca, R. F., and R. M. Galford. 2006. *Your Leadership Legacy: Why Looking Toward the Future Will Make You a Better Leader Today.* Boston: Harvard Business School Press.

Maxwell, J. C. 2008. *Leadership Gold.* Nashville, TN: Thomas Nelson.

Morris, L. 2011. "Top-Down Innovation: Leaders Define Innovative Culture." *RealInnovation.com.* Accessed April 18. www.realinnovation.com/content/c070528a.asp.

————. 2011. *The Innovation Master Plan: The CEO's Guide to Innovation.* Walnut Creek, CA: Innovation Academy.

Moss Kanter, R. 1997. *Rosabeth Moss Kanter on the Frontiers of Management.* Boston: Harvard Business Review Press.

Musselwhite, C. 2007. "Self Awareness and the Effective Leader." *Inc.* Published October 1. www.inc.com/resources/leadership/articles/20071001/musselwhite.html.

National Leadership Council, National Health Service. 2010. "What Is the LF?" *National Leadership Council.* Copyright 2010. http://nhsleadershipframework.rightmanagement.co.uk/what-is-the-lf.

Oden, S. 2009. "12 Leadership Legacy Traits—How Do You Measure Up?" *Synergistic Leadership.* Published February 25. http://synergisticleadership.wordpress.com/2009/02/25/12-leadership-legacy-traits-how-do-you-measure-up.

Parker, G. 2002. *Team Depot: A Warehouse of over 585 Tools to Reassess, Rejuvenate, and Rehabilitate Your Team.* San Francisco: Jossey-Bass.

Perry, F. 2001. *The Tracks We Leave: Ethics in Healthcare Management.* Chicago: Health Administration Press.

Quigley, W. 2011. "Working Through Differences." *Albuquerque Journal*, June 19, H1.

Robbins, H. 2007. "Leadership Skill: Leaving a Leadership Legacy." *harveyrobbins.com*. Published April 8. www.harveyrobbins.com/2007/04/08/leadership-skill-leaving-a-leadership-legacy/.

Sadler, W. A. 2000. *The Third Age: 6 Principles for Growth and Renewal After Forty.* Philadelphia: Perseus.

Sandstrom, J., and L. Smith. 2008. *Legacy Leadership: The Leader's Guide to Lasting Greatness.* Dallas, TX: CoachWorks Press.

Schulte, M. F. 2010. "Diversity in Healthcare: Leading Toward Culturally Competent Care." *Frontiers of Health Services Management* 26 (3): 1.

Schwartz, P. 1991. *The Art of the Long View.* New York: Doubleday.

Sloane, P. 2012. "Article Directory." *Destination Innovation.* Accessed May 10. www.destination-innovation.com/articles/.

Stein, S. J., D. Mann, P. Papadogiannis, and W. Gordon. 2009. *Emotional Intelligence Skills Assessment (EISA) Facilitator's Guide.* San Francisco: Pfeiffer.

Venegas, M. 2011. "Hispanics Must Use Growing Power Wisely." *Albuquerque Journal*, June 19, B3.

Watson, L. 2001. *How They Achieved: Stories of Personal Achievement and Business Success.* New York: Wiley & Sons.

Weil, A. 2005. *Healthy Aging.* New York: Random House

Weisman, R. 2003. "Harvard Raises Its Hand on Ethics: 1st-Year MBA Students Must Take New Course." *Boston Globe*, December 30, C1.

Weiss, R. S. 2005. *The Experience of Retirement.* Ithaca, NY: Cornell University Press.

Witt/Kieffer. 2007. "Inaugural Thought Leaders Forum." *Witt/Kieffer.* Accessed May 10, 2012. www.wittkieffer.com/file/thought-leadership/practice/Thought%20Leaders%20Forum%20White%20Paper%202008.pdf.

Zenger, J., and J. Folkman. 2002. *The Extraordinary Leader: Turning Good Managers into Great Leaders.* New York: McGraw-Hill.

Interviewed Leaders

Brian Campion, MD, is senior fellow in healthcare leadership at Opus College of Business, University of St. Thomas, in Minneapolis.

Ed Dahlberg, LFACHE, is former president and CEO of St. Luke's Regional Medical Center in Boise, Idaho.

Thomas C. Dolan, PhD, FACHE, CAE, is president and CEO of the American College of Healthcare Executives in Chicago.

Martin L. "Chip" Doordan, LFACHE, is CEO emeritus at Anne Arundel Health System in Annapolis, Maryland.

David J. Fine, FACHE, is president and CEO of St. Luke's Episcopal Health System in Houston.

Patricia Gabow, MD, is CEO of Denver (Colorado) Health & Hospital Authority.

Patrick G. Hays, FACHE, is an advisor to management at the University of Southern California in Los Angeles.

Paul B. Hofmann, DrPH, FACHE, is president of Hofmann Healthcare Group in Moraga, California.

Stanley F. Hupfeld is chairman of INTEGRIS Family of Foundations at INTEGRIS Health in Oklahoma City.

John G. King, LFACHE, is president of John G. King Associates in Scottsdale, Arizona.

Lowell C. Kruse, LFACHE, is president and CEO emeritus at Heartland Health in St. Joseph, Missouri.

Stephanie S. McCutcheon, FACHE, is principal at McCutcheon and Co. in Pasadena, Maryland.

Stanley R. Nelson, LFACHE, is chairman of Scottsdale Institute in Minneapolis.

Kirk Oglesby is president emeritus of AnMed Health in Anderson, South Carolina.

Samuel L. Ross, MD, is CEO of Bon Secours Baltimore (Maryland) Health System.

Nancy M. Schlichting is CEO of Henry Ford Health System in Detroit.

William C. Schoenhard, FACHE, is deputy under secretary for Health Operations and Management at the US Department of Veterans Affairs in Washington, D.C.

Harvey Smith is president and CEO of Pacific Medical Centers in Seattle.

Mark R. Tolosky, JD, FACHE, is president and CEO of Baystate Health in Springfield, Massachusetts.

Gail L. Warden, LFACHE, is president emeritus of Henry Ford Health System in Detroit.

Donald C. Wegmiller, FACHE, is vice chairman of Scottsdale Institute and chairman emeritus of Integrated Healthcare Strategies in Minneapolis.

Index

Fine, David J.: on diversity, 72, 75, 77, 84, 88, 95; on ethics, 41
Folkman, Joseph, 35
Followers, 55–56, 60
Freedman, Marc, 128–129, 130, 131, 134

Gabow, Patricia, 58, 111
Gender, and diversity, 77, 83–85, 147
General Electric (GE), 107
Generation gap/divide, 85–87
George, Bill: on ethics, 35, 40; on integrity/character, 25; on self-awareness, 17, 19–20; on values, 26, 33
Gere, Richard, 136–137
Ghandi, Indira, 84
Glass ceiling, 84
Globalization: and ethics, 26; and diversity, 71, 75
Goldsmith, Marshall, 52, 53–54
Good to Great (Collins), 11, 34
Grandparenting, 134, 137–139, *138*

Hanberg, Bob, 60
Handy, Charles, 131–132
Hanson, Kirk, 61
Harvard Business School, 33
Harvard University, 136
Hays, Patrick G.: on diversity, 76, 78, 85, 90, 97; on ethics, 32; on innovation, 110; on retirement, 128, 131
Healing the Divide (charity), 136
Health Research & Educational Trust (HRET), 97, 100
Henry Ford Health System, 73
Hispanics, and diversity in healthcare, 80, 82
Hofmann, Paul B., 26, 38, 79–80, 93, 99
Houghton, Armory, 34

HRET. *See* Health Research & Educational Trust
Humility, 6, 11, 12, 19, 21, 34
Hupfeld, Stanley F., 7

Idea scouts, 102
IFD. *See* Institute for Diversity in Health Management
IMGs. *See* International medical graduates
Immigration, 73
Impact Awards, 136
"Improving Access to Services for Persons with Limited Language Proficiency" (Executive Order 13166), 98
Innovation, 101–112, 147–148; key actions for legacy road map, 112; and celebration culture, 121; labs and culture, 106–108; leadership, 101–103; milestones, 108–111; networks, 107–108, *109*; social, 103; unleashing, 103–106
Innovational wisdom, 101
Institute for Diversity in Health Management (IFD), 97, 100
Institute of Medicine, 71, 81, 83
Integrated Healthcare Strategies, 54
Integrity, 25, 27–28, 34, 39, 44, 59, 145; key actions for legacy road map, 45; and celebration culture, 122. *See also* Ethics
International Health Leadership Program, 52, 119
International Labor Rights Fund, 75
International medical graduates (IMGs), 76, 88, 90

James, Henry, 140
Jobs, Steve, 111
Joint Commission, 82, 98

About the Authors

Frankie Perry, RN, LFACHE, has held senior positions in both nursing and hospital administration. She served as assistant medical center director of Hurley Medical Center in Flint, Michigan, for several years. In addition to her hospital experience, she served as executive vice president of the American College of Healthcare Executives (ACHE) and as a national and international healthcare consultant with engagements in Cairo, Egypt; Doha, Qatar; and Mumbai, among others. She is a well-published author of articles on ethics and healthcare management and was a 1984 recipient of the Edgar A. Hayhow Award for Article of the Year awarded by ACHE. Her book *The Tracks We Leave: Ethics in Healthcare Management*, was published in 2001 by Health Administration Press, and *Management Mistakes in Healthcare: Identification, Correction and Prevention*, co-authored with Paul B. Hofmann, DrPH, FACHE, was published by Cambridge University Press in 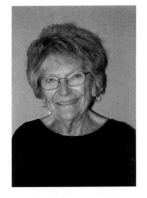 2005. She currently serves as adjunct faculty for the University of New Mexico. In addition, she teaches an online seminar, "Management Mistakes, Moral Dilemmas and Lessons Learned," for ACHE. In 2008, she was the recipient of a Regent's Award and, in 2011, she received the Lifetime Service Award, both awarded by ACHE. She is a past member of the board of directors for the Commission for the Accreditation of Health Care Management Education.

James A. Rice, PhD, is an internationally recognized authority on healthcare policy, governance, and strategy development. He is director of a large international leadership development program with Management Science for Health. Dr. Rice also serves as vice chairman of The Governance Institute. He holds faculty positions at Cambridge University and the Program in Health Administration at the University of Minnesota's School of Public Health.

At Integrated Healthcare Strategies, he led the Governance & Leadership Services practice, focusing his consulting work on strategic governance, visioning for health sector and not-for-profit 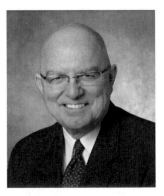 organizations, leadership development for physicians, strategic capital financial planning, mergers and acquisitions, and enterprise risk management analyses for physician–hospital joint ventures.

Prior to these positions, Dr. Rice was a senior officer of the largest integrated healthcare system in Minnesota. He has also worked with numerous US arts organizations, colleges, and universities on governance and strategy development.

Dr. Rice has authored articles in publications such as *Modern Healthcare*, *Trustee*, the *Harvard Business Review*, and the *Journal of Health Administration*. He has lectured extensively on health policy issues, governance, and strategic planning, and he has conducted board retreats across the United States.

Among Dr. Rice's awards, he has received the University of Minnesota School of Public Health Distinguished Alumni Leadership Award, a National Institute of Health doctoral fellowship, and the American Hospital Association's Corning Award for excellence in hospital planning. He is a member of the American College of Healthcare Executives and a Fellow of Health and Life Sciences Partnership in London. Dr. Rice holds master's and doctoral degrees in management and health policy from the University of Minnesota.